EVERYTHING YOU NEED TO KNOW ABOUT FAT LOSS...

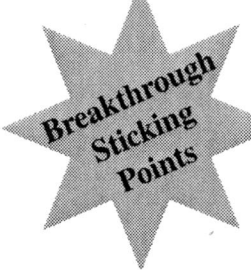

Breakthrough Sticking Points

RE-CHARGE Your Metabolism

By
Chris Aceto

The objective of this book is to inform and educate. It is not intended as a prescription or substitute for health care by a professional.

ISBN 0-9669168-2-4

First Printing - May 1997
Second Printing - May 1998
Third Printing - March 1999
Fourth Printing - March 2000

Printed in the United States by
Morris Publishing
3212 East Highway 30
Kearney, NE 68847
1-800-650-7888

TABLE OF CONTENTS

Chapter One

Everything You Need To Know On Weight Loss

Why another book about weight loss, losing body fat, and diet? Surely, there are enough! Just peruse your local book super store, and you will soon become overwhelmed with the amount of books guiding, prescribing, and selling the latest tips, info, research, ideas, potions, pills and promises pertaining to losing fat.

I find much of the weight loss information to be conflicting, confusing, overwhelming, and ultimately can do more harm than good. For example, we have the "rice diet" and the "fruit diet." Some say fruit turns to fat while others only eat fruits before noon. Fruit can turn to fat compared to what, donuts? I think not! I never saw anyone sit down and eat too much fruit, say 3 apples a pear and a banana. However, we've all, at some time or another, sat down in front of the TV and gobbled down a whole pizza, or a box of cookies, or a mound of ice cream. Is fruit fattening? You're smart, you tell me. For those who prescribe eating fruit only before noon, I say this, "What if you work the late shift and do not wake up until noon, then what?"

Of course, the low fat diet, the incredible dietary revelation started by Pritikin works. Or does it? The low fat approach to losing weight prescribes lowering your intake of dietary fat to less than 10% of your total calories. The food industry has responded by making nearly every food product available with no fat or little fat added. Now, we can eat fat free pretzels, fat free potato chips, fat free ice cream, fat free pizza, fat free tuna sandwiches, fat free cookies, and the list continues. My question is this. With so much to choose from, why are we Americans, on average, fatter than ever?

Some weight loss books blame your laziness. The authors of these books sound something like this. "Exercise, burns calories, so performing enough exercise will keep a person lean or promote fat loss in everyone." Sorry. While exercise can help, it is not the full story, the end all. What you eat, the amount of total calories you eat, and the types of foods you eat also has an effect on fat storage. Some people can get very lean with exercise, but others should rely more on diet. Furthermore, there are more gyms, health clubs, resorts, personal trainers, exercise machines, and gadgets than ever. So what's the scoop? How is it, we are fatter than ever? Sure, there are lots of awesome and incredible bodies around, but as a whole, the population is pretty sloppy. I know we are failing the fat test when I consistently see fat kids at malls, schools, and church. Sure there were some chunky kids around when I was young. Every school had its fat little kid who was the brunt of jokes and picked on, but there are so many now!

There are fat loss pills, creams, drinks, gurus,

prescription pills, appetite suppressants, and therapy. There's late night infomercials, gadgets, clinics, medical weight loss programs, Jenny Craig, Weight Watchers, Slimfast, MetRx, Ensure. And if that is not enough, we are bombarded with stars, who have always appeared lean, fit and trim, hocking everything from a thigh toning machine to an indoor roller blading device. I am sure you've seen those ab machines on T.V. too. I'll let you in on a secret. First, the models used for the ab machines probably never in their lives used these machines. Second, the infomercials imply you will be able to achieve some awesome looking abs by using the ab machine. I highly doubt that would occur. To get the abs the model has, you would need to eat the right diet to strip away all the fat covering the abdominal region to allow the abs to shine. Next, you would have to build the abdominals with exercise.

P.T Barnum was the founder to the phrase, "There is a sucker born every minute." This was true in his day, and still holds true today. Let me tell you how crazy the diet and exercise industry is. A few years ago, I had a meeting with a very prominent publisher of an exercise magazine. Over a business lunch, he told me, "Chris, if you want to make money, you should write a diet book, but not just any old diet and exercise book. Take an odd approach, make it really gimmicky and outrageous. Promise overnight transformations, promise instant results, promise the reader that this diet is top secret, one used by Hollywood stars and top professional bodybuilders. Tell the reader you consult with Pro Athletes, movie stars, even politicians." As I grew skeptical and as my feeling of respect for this individual suddenly began to change as he spoke, he added, "The crazier the promises sound, the more people will buy. The buying public is just so damn naive, confused and desperate, they'll try anything!" After that conversation, I called my wife and we agreed that if I ever wrote a book, it would be the exact opposite of the rich publisher's recommendation . . . .

Chapter Two

History of Fat Loss

It is common sense and obvious to me people have been dieting since the invention of the mirror. Vanity is nothing new, it simply has become magnified over time.

Today experts tell us lean people live longer and are more productive in their daily lives. For this reason, millions have embarked upon some sort of weight loss program. Although millions diet and exercise to live longer or to feel better and have more energy, my guess is the majority do so to look better. We aspire to the lean image portrayed by those we see on television, in print ads, and in movies.

Years ago, people who wanted to lose fat did so based upon a very limited amount of information. Before the invention of the word "calorie" people lost weight by fasting. Fasting was introduced to mankind by god. The jews fast, as do the Christians, and muslims. All do so because god told the prophets that abstaining from food was good for the soul as well as the physical body. A common physical change that all three groups noticed was a loss in weight, a decrease in body fat. Thus, to lose weight, the first dieter would abstain from food and drink water. It was then, and is today, a proven way to lose fat, albeit an extreme approach.

When a person abstains from food, the body has to break down body tissue to use for survival. Most of this fuel comes from stored energy in the form of body fat reserves. Unfortunately, a severe fast also is a dangerous fast as the body also calls upon other tissues to be used as fuel. With fasting, the body chooses a mixture of stored body fat as fuel and lean body mass. Lean body mass is readily tapped as fuel. Just as the body taps body fat and breaks it down to use it as energy, it can do the same with muscle and organs. When deprived of food, the body can easily break down the heart, the liver, and other organs to make fuel. The body will also rip apart the muscles throughout the body to make fuel during a starvation fast. While fat is burned up quickly as fuel, muscle and organs are also burned. This can lead to exhaustion and eventually death. So, we can conclude, the fast, while spiritually advantageous, isn't exactly the smartest approach to losing fat.

Once people figured out prolonged fasting worked, but the negative was death, they began to alter the fasting approach to weight loss. Thus, the modified fast was born. The modified fast involved abstaining from food completely for as long as you could, and when you finally broke down, your willpower crushed and your appetite screaming in high gear, you would eat. Some would eat a small amount and drink a ton of water to suppress the appetite, but others would go crazy, break down, and eat as if it was their last meal on earth, probably negating any fat lost during a few days of fasting.

With the breakthroughs in science, man "discovered" the calorie and the never ending task of tabulating numbers, keeping records, and avoiding large portions began. However, the dieter did not know how many calories he required in a day, so in hopes of losing fat, and with little knowledge, he resorted to a method that is still prevalent today. That method is, "If you are not sure how many calories you should be eating to lose weight, just take the conservative route, and eat less." For many, the magical number of 1000 seemed to be low enough to work, and many who followed a diet that yielded only 1000 calories in a day lost weight.

Many who chose the 1000 calorie a day approach soon discovered what scientists would prove many years later, the dreaded dieting plateau. Science has shown that when calories are restricted, the body compensates by obtaining energy from stored body fat. But, as calories remain low for an extended period of time, the body makes another adaptive response. With prolonged calorie restriction or with severe calorie restriction, the body will begin to conserve calories. In time the 1000 calorie approach fails because the body, not wanting to die as happens in a severe and long fast, but having enough calories to survive, will make the most out of the 1000 calories by radically slowing down the rate at which it burns those 1000 calories. The result is fat is lost on a very low calorie approach, but the diet ultimately ceases to work like it did in the beginning.

Early research into metabolism and nutrition revealed many physiological understandings that dieters tried to use to enable them to lose fat. From day one, dieters have realized that eating less leads to weight loss. However, astute dieters realized the limitations of the 1000 calorie diet. Research began to prove that with a caloric restriction, body protein, specifically in the form of muscle mass was also being shed along with body fat. To combat this, dieters put a simple twist to the 1000 calorie diet. They ate all the calories from protein foods. The idea was simple. Count calories and limit the total to 1000, but eat only protein foods. The 1000 calories is low enough to cause the body to shed fat and eating more protein would prevent the body from using muscle as fuel. The mind set was simple. Flood the body with extra protein foods like meats, cheese, pork, hamburg, and chicken, but limit the caloric intake. The extra protein will keep the body from tapping muscle as fuel since it has the raw material or protein it needs in the foods. This worked better than fasting but it lacked variety and was just too difficult to maintain even for those who had the greatest willpower.

Around the early 1900's, scientists began looking into the reason why people overate. Scientists realized if people ate less, they would lose weight. Thus began the search for effective diet pills. The first diet pills focused on suppressing the appetite so less food would be consumed. Inventions like benzocaine were common. Placed upon the tongue, benzocaine would dull the taste buds and leave a tingling and weird sensation in the mouth which scientists hoped would suppress the appetite. It worked for some, and failed for others. Similar success probably could be reached by washing your mouth out with soap every time you felt hungry. Surely, any foul substance that alters the sense of taste could keep a person from eating, no matter what the substance.

Other approaches included suppressing the appetite by stimulating the brain. This was initially accomplished with the administration of amphetamines - speed. Speed seems to suppress appetite by stimulating the appetite center of the brain. Plus, it fights fatigue by stimulating the nervous system. So far, it sounds like a monumental discovery and aid for dieters. You lose weight by eating less and you have plenty of energy. Unfortunately, as with many drugs, they work too good. Over stimulating the nervous system can lead to many maladies like schizophrenia, paranoia, irritability, inability to think clearly, and total exhaustion. Other drugs have been developed to decrease the appetite. Most exert strong stimulatory effects upon the nervous system but are much safer than pure speed. These drugs are similar to speed in their ability to suppress the appetite though they have been altered to have lesser overall body stimulating effects. Therefore, they are believed to be much safer. I will discuss many of them in the Chapter 15 on drugs.

At one time, drugs to increase the amount of calories burned were popular among the medical profession. Thyroid hormones govern the amount of energy the body uses in any given day. Supplemental thyroid could increase the metabolic rate but the body can readily adapt to the artificially high amounts of thyroid a patient is using. In healthy individuals, the body releases thyroid hormone into the blood and this is converted into a more active form that the body tissues use. When a patient, in hopes of shedding fat, swallows thyroid medication, the body eventually responds and adapts by slowing the conversion of the artificial hormone to the more active form in the body. Furthermore, the body's own release of this hormone is suppressed. Any increase in metabolism does not last. Those who try to drastically increase thyroid medication to force the body to increase the metabolism, ultimately fail, as high amounts of thyroid will exert effects similar to a modified fast. Fat is lost but muscle tissue and organs are destroyed and broken down to be used as fuel.

Scientists soon discovered a special phenomena that occurs with food intake called thermogenesis. Thermogenesis is a fancy word for heat. Foods are really forms of energy. When food is eaten the body breaks down the fuel from the foods to obtain this energy to maintain life and to do work. The fate of this energy is three fold. Energy can be used up by the body, it can be stored as muscle glycogen to be used at a later date or it can be stored as body fat. The third fate of energy derived from food is it can be "wasted as heat." The body is always producing heat, much like a furnace. When foods are consumed the body temperature rises and some of the calories from the foods we eat are simply burned off as heat leaving less "net" calories available for the body, the muscle cells and fat cells. Some foods exert a strong thermic effect while others do not. Specifically, protein foods exert the greatest thermic effect. Roughly 20% of the calories derived from protein foods are not available to be used by the body because they are burned off as body heat. Of course, dieters adopted this fact, and once again, protein became the dieter's choice food. People ate a lot

14

of protein hoping it would have a thermogenic "over-drive" effect. As with any diet that is lower in calories, the approach worked to some degree, mainly due to a total lower caloric intake.

Over time, as dieters failed in their quest for a lean body, psychologists postulated the theory that people overeat or under eat due to their emotional state. Some studies showed a correlation between depression and overeating. Psychologists reasoned a person could only free themselves from overeating with intensive therapy. Once the underlying psychological problem was found and treated, a patient would resume eating normally. While therapy may be helpful for some, it did not accommodate the fact that millions are overweight who seem to be perfectly content in their lives, and many can not lose weight who have undertaken years of exhaustive therapy.

To some degree, I have been involved and infatuated with body fat control for 15 years. Diets come and go. The Rice Diet, The Fruit Diet, The Low Carb Diet, The High Carb Diet, The High Fat Diet, The Low Fat Diet, The Fiber Diet, and the list continues. What each and every diet has in common is a controlled caloric intake. One thing we know for sure, when calories are reduced, the body calls upon other sources for fuel, one of them is stored body fat. So, unlike others who say, "Diets do not work," I disagree and say, "All diets do work!" The problem is this. They are either difficult to maintain for long periods of time, or they do not supply enough calories, so a discouraged dieter usually throws in the towel and quits.

My first diet was usurped from my sister. She lost a

lot of weight, and I didn't like the way I looked and thought I would feel better by shedding some excess fat. Like any dieter, the only information I knew was "calories." Calories, my sister told me, caused body fat to accumulate. Being young and naive, I set out to rid myself of calories. I stopped eating, save for an egg and one piece of toast for breakfast, nothing for lunch, and salad and chicken for dinner. I quickly lost 13 pounds. I felt great when I could fit into clothes that were previously too snug, but became exhausted and just damn irritable and mean. The diet ceased being a diet when I broke down and obliterated myself with an un-ending stream of food: cookies, ice cream, cake, pizza, etc., all in a period of 6 hours. I felt so mad, discouraged, and upset. Instead of getting right back on the diet that was severe, but was accomplishing what I wanted, I gained 15 pounds in a few weeks by eating relatively normal. Now, two pounds fatter than when I started my first diet, I began to strategize. I needed a new diet - a better one. Everywhere I looked from the newspaper to magazines, to the library and bookstores, I found plenty on the confusing topic of weight loss. I purchased all of it. I read everything. I reasoned I would absorb and digest every bit of info out there on diet and become an authority! Surely, if I read everything available pertaining to the subject of weight loss, I could figure out or find the best diets and disregard the bad ones. Well, in doing so, I became more confused, as I am sure many of you are right now.

Chapter Three

Calories

Calories are a measuring unit-a way to measure how much energy is produced from foods. We need calories, as fuel, to think. The brain will die without sugar. Our heart needs fuel from calories to work, to pump blood throughout the body. All the organs need fuel to perform their specific jobs. Just sitting in bed all day long without getting up and without moving requires a very large amount of calories. These calories are needed to maintain the organs in the body so that they can function properly. Any activity on top of sitting in bed all day requires additional calories.

Typing, driving to work, giving a presentation at your job, shuttling the kids around town, and other small physical tasks all require additional calories.

Your muscles require fuel to perform work. Walking requires calories. If the walk becomes harder, the body needs more calories and if the walk becomes a run, even more calories are needed. The harder the work, the more calories you need. The point is this. Calories are a good thing, not a bad thing. You need calories to live and to do work. It is an excess caloric intake that can lead to fat storage. Fat storage is nothing more than a bank for calories. When too many calories are ingested, the bank opens up to save those calories for a later time. This bank will hold these calories until there is a shortage. When a shortage of calories occurs, the bank will release some of its stores so the body can survive or perform work.

Unfortunately, when the bank already has deposits, and more calories are consumed, above and beyond what the body needs for survival and to perform work in any one day, the bank pays a "dividend" in the form of more fat storage.

Most people who follow a diet have absolutely no idea how many calories they need. From above we know the body needs calories just to maintain its organs and muscle mass. Organs and muscle require calories while at rest - when you are doing nothing at all. This number is far greater than most people believe. Body fat does not require calories. There are many ways to find out how many calories an individual needs in any one day. There are several complicated formulas, but I use a simple one. Here it is.

Finding Resting* Caloric Needs
1) Weigh yourself
2) Find Body Fat Percentage (calipers are accurate)
3) Take your Lean Body Mass
     (total weight in pounds - fat weight in pounds)
4) Add a zero

Example
1) My weight is 200 pounds
2) My Body Fat is 10%
3) which means my Lean Body Mass is 180
   (200-20)
4) 180 + 0 = 1800

From the formula above, I can estimate I need roughly 1800 calories a day. My organs and muscles require I supply it with 1800 calories each day just to maintain a normal and healthy body. If I do anything, go to work, visit friends, go to the mall for a stroll or exercise, I need more calories to fuel these activities. Therefore, I can summarize 1800 calories is the lowest level I can reduce my calories in any day. Reducing below 1800 is unhealthy and dangerous. Furthermore, it is absolutely impossible to obtain all the micronutrients (vitamins and minerals) I need from such fewer calories.

As you can see, the more lean body mass one has, the more calories needed at rest. Eight hundred calorie diets or even 1200 calorie diets are just too few. Even a small person has more than 80 pounds of lean body mass and will require much more than 800 calories a day (80 + 0 = 800).

Types of Calories

Calories are derived from foods and there are three types or sub groups of calories. They are carbohydrates, proteins, and fat.

Carbohydrates are derived from non animal foods.

Examples are rice, pasta, beans, breads, potatoes, yams, fruits, and anything that contains sugar. *All carbohydrate foods eventually are broken down and absorbed as sugar.* Technically, there is no difference in the final result from eating rice or potatoes or candy. All three will enter the blood as sugar.

The body keeps a tight check on the amount of sugar in the blood. For the body to function normally, sugar levels must stay normal or stable between 70 mg/100 ml to 110 mg/100 ml of blood. The carbohydrate foods a person eats enter the blood as sugar, thereby affecting how much sugar is in the blood.

I have established that I need 1800 calories a day at rest, with absolutely no activity. If I eat 1800 calories a day, my body will be able to maintain the normal blood sugar parameter of 70 to 110. The body will use these calories to maintain my organs and muscle.

When more calories are eaten then I need, in this case carbohydrate calories, the amount of sugar in the blood rises. When blood sugar levels rise, the body will store some of the carbohydrates to be used later, in case there is a shortage of calories, especially carbohydrates. When sugar levels in the blood rise as a result of eating above your caloric needs or from eating excess carbohydrates, the excess is stored in the liver and the muscle as liver and muscle glycogen.

The liver and muscle can store a limited amount of carbohydrates. If blood sugar levels rise or approach 110 and if caloric content exceeds the daily requirement a person needs, all extra carbohydrates will be stored as fat.

When calories, especially carbohydrates are curtailed, the amount of sugar in the blood drops. When this occurs, the body demands that the liver or muscle, the two backup storage areas for carbohydrates, break down their carbohydrate reserves and shunt the carbohydrates back into the blood to keep the normal level of 70 to 110. If blood sugar levels stay low, close to 70, and if too few calories are consumed, the body will also start to use more body fat as fuel.

Protein

Protein is derived from animal foods: chicken, turkey, meats, lamb, fish, and all dairy products. Protein supplies the building blocks for life - amino acids. When you eat protein foods, the body breaks the food down into amino acids, in a way similar to the body breaking down carbohydrates into sugar.

Amino acids are used for thousands - probably millions - of reactions in the body. In a diet that lacks protein, the body will quickly begin to look for amino acids to maintain life. If there are far too few amino acids in the blood, the body will make amino acids at a life-threatening cost. Amino acids will be derived, stripped really, from organs and muscle. Both organs and muscle are made of protein. The body can destroy its own organs and muscle just to keep a balanced level of amino acids in the blood. The nonactive body needs roughly 1 gram of protein for every two pounds of lean body mass, at rest. Therefore, I need a MINIMUM of

90 grams of protein a day (180 lb. LBM/2 = 90) while doing nothing but staying at home and not leaving my bed.

If carbohydrate intake is too low, and calorie requirements are below a minimum (1800 for me) the body will convert some protein to sugar. Basically, if sugar levels are too low, and liver and muscle glycogen stores are also low in sugar, the body will readily manufacture sugar from amino acids.

Very Low Protein Diet

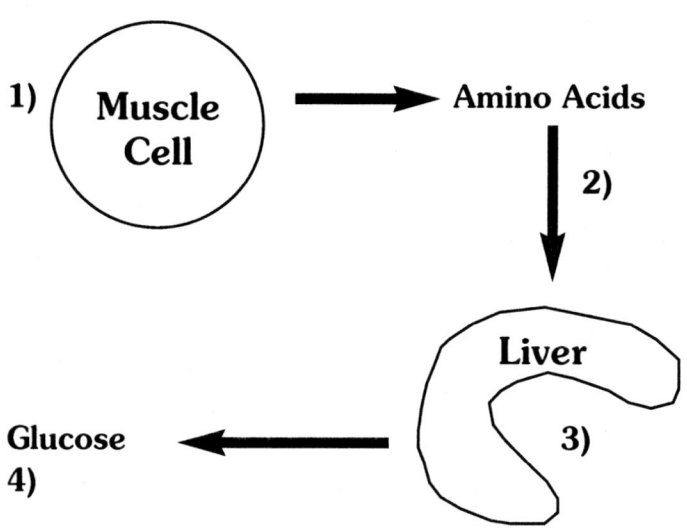

1) Muscles breakdown and release amino acids
2) Amino Acids are sent to the liver
3) Liver changes amino acids into glucose (sugar)
4) Glucose enters blood from the liver

Result: Muscle Wastage!!

Many people believe protein can not be stored as fat. This is untrue, as all three macronutrients, carbohydrates, fat, and protein can all be stored as fat. Protein undeservingly earned this reputation because it has a higher thermic rate than both carbohydrates and fat. Of the three, protein creates the most heat in the body. Roughly 15% to 20% of the protein calories you eat will be burned off as heat leaving 80% of the calories you eat available to be broken down into amino acids to be used by the body. Therefore, a piece of fish yielding 200 calories of protein will, in reality, yield only 160 to 170 calories in the body.

Fats

Dietary fats have the greatest reputation as a fat storer. Americans count fat grams like a tight wad counts money. However, there is more to fat loss than simply counting up fat grams. That's not to say counting fat grams is a bad idea. Each gram of fat yields 9 calories while each gram of carbohydrates or each gram of protein yields only four calories. So, it is easy to see why many count fat grams. Gram for gram, fat yields more than double the amount of calories that the same amount of protein or carbohydrates yield.

One reason many cut out fat grams is to radically reduce calorie intake without cutting back on total food volume. For example, 8 ounces of chicken breast yields 200 calories while the exact same amount of chicken thighs yields approximately 300 calories. Frying foods adds huge amounts of calories. My wife makes oven "fried" french fries. One cup yields 120 calories but one cup of real french fries yields 240 calories.

Sugar: The Nitty Gritty

OK, we already talked about carbohydrates. Now I'll be specific. All carbohydrate foods enter the blood as glucose, a sugar also referred to as blood sugar. Glucose stimulates the pancreas to release a special storage hormone called insulin. Insulin is responsible for regulating how much sugar can stay in the blood. If there is a lot of glucose in the blood, the body outputs a lot of insulin. If there is very little glucose in the blood, the body will output a smaller amount of insulin. Insulin has three effects. Insulin clears sugar from the blood and deposits it into tissues. The tissues are liver, muscle and fat. The first two locations are good, the latter is bad news to the person seeking a lean body.

There are two kinds of carbohydrates. Simple carbohydrates are sugars known as monosaccharides. They are found in fruits, fruit juices, honey, jellies, jams, and in table sugar and soda. The other carbohydrates, known as complex carbohydrates, are nothing more than simple carbohydrates linked together to form complex or longer chain carbohydrates. Complex carbohydrates can elicit less insulin release than simple carbohydrates. Simple carbohydrates are broken down, digested and absorbed with ease and speed. The result is the sugar enters the blood stream quickly and the body perceives an abundance of sugar in the blood at one time. It reacts by trying to deal with the situation. Lots of sugar in the blood stream or a concentrated amount of sugar at one time causes the pancreas to output more insulin. Compare this to the reaction that occurs when complex carbohydrates are eaten. Some common complex carbohydrates that you probably like to eat are potatoes, yams, wild rice, pasta, beans, and whole grain bread. These carbohydrates are broke down slower (see chart below) than simple sugars because the body must first cleave the long chain and take one sugar at a time off of the complex link of simple sugars that make up the complex carbohydrate. Then, the sugar link that has been broken from the longer chain enters the blood stream.

Carbohydrate Breakdown

Simple Carbohydrates

◯ = Mono Saccharide

Complex Carbohydrates

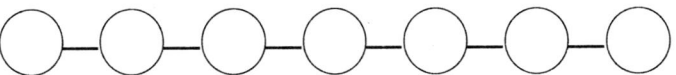

Digestion of Complex Carbohydrates

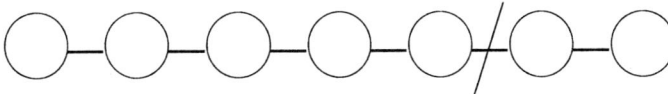

Disaccharide

Mono Saccharide

The difference between simple sugars and complex sugars (complex carbohydrates) is the speed at which they enter the blood as glucose and the total amount of insulin that is released. Here's an easy example. Compare 200 calories of fruit juice to 200 calories of potatoes. Although the calories are the same, one will produce a larger release of insulin than another. The juice, comprised of simple sugar, will enter the blood faster causing a quick accumulation of sugar in the blood. The body will output insulin to lower the amount of sugar in the blood, closer to normal levels of 70 to 110. When 200 calories of potatoes is eaten, the body must break down each small link of sugar that makes up the complex chain. Therefore, the sugar enters the blood at a slower rate. Compared to the sugar in the fruit juice, the sugar in the potatoes breaks down slower. Since less sugar is in the blood all at once, the body reacts by releasing a smaller amount of insulin to deal with the smaller amount of sugar.

However, all complex carbohydrates are not always better choices as a carbohydrate source. Fruits contain fructose, a special sugar that does not require insulin to be used by the body. Fruits are definitely a good food and a smart choice for the weight conscious as it is very low in calories.

Complex carbohydrates can also cause a large output in insulin. When too many carbohydrates are eaten at one meal, the carbohydrates dump a lot of sugar into the blood. When this happens, the body will clear the abundant amount of sugar out of the blood by releasing lots of insulin to deal with the excessive sugar. *High insulin favors fat storage.*

The Fiber Connection

Many claim that fiber is a good tool in weight control. I agree. Fiber acts with sugar by slowing the release of carbohydrates from the gut. If food from the gut is released at a slower rate, then digestion is slower, and ultimately, the sugar in carbohydrates are released slower into the blood. When sugar is released at a slower rate in the blood, less insulin is released. Mashed potatoes are a poor choice for weight loss compared to the exact same calorie and carbohydrate content found in a baked potato. The mashed potatoes lack fiber and will enter the blood as sugar faster than a baked potato.

Fiber also has been shown to make people feel fuller than those who do not eat fiber. Fiber adds texture and taste without adding calories. Specifically, fiber is a "non-digestible" food substance. Many call it a carbohydrate but that is inaccurate. They do so because fiber is common in complex carbohydrates. Fiber can not be broken down by the body. It simply passes right through the human digestive tract adding no calories. Eating 100 calories of broccoli yields zero calories to the body. In fact, it takes some digestive energy to pass the vegetables through the body, so the net calorie contribution of most vegetables is negative! Vegetables like corn and peas do provide calories, complex carbohydrates. The carbohydrate the body uses is inside the skins. The outer layer passes right through the body as it is made of fiber.

Fiber is found in vegetables, whole grain bread, not those pseudo wheat breads at the grocery store that seem to be as light as air and foods found in nature, not "made" by man. Fiber rich natural foods include potatoes, yams, brown rice, bulgur, oats as in slow cooking oatmeal, beans, roots like yucca, all fruits and grains. We eat very few of these foods. Instead we opt for white bread, crackers, pasta made from white flour, white flour products in general, white rice, soda, fruit juice, sugar drinks like TANG or Sunny Delite that masquerade as fruit juice, candy, ice cream, crackers, etc . . . Refined foods that lack fiber can elicit a greater release of insulin than foods that naturally retain fiber. The result: the U.S. population is fatter than ever.

Sugar, Insulin, and Fat Storage

So far, I have presented to you the way the body handles sugar from carbohydrates. Specifically, I have focused on insulin. Now I want to draw your attention to the other effects, both positive and negative, of this potent hormone.

High insulin is caused by high amounts of sugar in the blood. High amount of sugar will be present in the blood stream when a person simply eats a lot of carbohydrates, even if those carbohydrates are from a high fiber, "healthy" natural source. High insulin levels will also be present when one consumes sugar laden carbs, juices, or simple carbs in general.

We also know the role of insulin. It clears sugar from the blood to bring the concentration of sugar in the blood back to a normal level of 70 to 110. When insulin clears sugar from the blood, it will try to place this sugar into reserves to be used at a later time. The three reserve locations for excess sugar is the liver, muscles, and fat stores. When liver and muscle stores are full, all excess sugar will be placed in fat stores. When there is still room in liver and muscle stores for sugar, the excess sugar in the blood, from eating carbohydrates, will be stored in the muscle or liver.

However, high insulin levels can cause the sugar to be stored in both places muscle/liver AND fat cells even if liver and muscle stores for sugar are not full! This may explain why a person who skips a lot of meals, and does not overeat, but consumes a moderate calorie diet, can gain fat by eating refined foods and sugar foods. Although calories are not excessive, insulin levels are high due to the wrong food choices, or eating too much at one meal. Fat is constantly being stored.

High insulin levels also affect appetite. Rats injected with insulin will eat until their stomachs explode while rats that have the pancreas (which makes insulin) removed, will starve to death because they refuse to eat. Insulin, in high amounts, is an appetite stimulant.

High insulin also exerts an interesting metabolic effect. When insulin levels are high they exert a special effect on fat cells. High insulin release causes the release of an enzyme called lipoprotein lipase (LPL). LPL retards the fat cell from breaking down to be used as fuel. The body always uses a mixture of fuel sources when at rest. Primarily fat is used to fuel a resting body. Some of this fat comes from dietary fat, the fat we eat in our foods and some comes from fat storage. If insulin levels are high all the time due to excessive calories, or low fiber food choices, or the inclusion of simple carbohydrates, the fat cell will not be used as fuel. Even those who do aerobics, in hopes of losing fat, will find weight loss to be very difficult if the diet is not adjusted to control insulin output.

The pancreas that is responsible for releasing insulin also releases an opposing hormone called glucagon. It's job is similar to insulin - to keep blood sugar levels normal, between 70 and 110. When carbohydrates are lacking in the diet, glucagon is released. Glucagon calls upon both the liver and muscles, storage cites for carbohydrates, to provide glucose. Glucagon stimulates the muscles and liver to send sugar back to the blood whenever sugar levels become too low. We can say that glucagon "opposes" insulin. Although both help the body to keep blood sugar levels in check, insulin is a "storer" of sugar while glucagon "liberates" sugar. Likewise, insulin promotes the increase of lipoprotein lipase that causes fat cells to stay full of fat, but glucagon allows fat to be broken down. Glucagon releases the enzyme, hormone sensitive lipase (HSL) which works on fat cells. HSL allows fat cells to be broken down to be used as fuel.

The body is always releasing both insulin and glucagon. After a meal that is made of protein and carbohydrates insulin is the primary hormone released, although glucagon can be released simultaneously, yet in small amounts. Between meals, when sugar levels in the blood begin to fall, glucagon comes into play. A high carbohydrate intake in a diet that provides too many calories will release so much insulin that the insulin will override any fat and sugar liberating effect.

A moderate calorie diet that includes lots of sugar will do the same. The net effect is sugar will be cleared from the blood with the help of insulin. Some sugar will be deposited in fat cells and the higher amount of insulin will block fat release from fat cells. Eat protein with your carbohydrates to release glucagon which can offset some fat storing effects of insulin.

Dietary Fats: **The Body Fat Connection**

Dietary fat is the third macronutrient. The other two are protein and carbohydrates. Americans are appalled by fat yet do not completely understand it's role in human nutrition.

Fats are disliked and discarded by most weight conscious individuals because it provides double the amount of calories, gram for gram, when compared to either carbohydrates or protein. As America has become fatter, it's intake of dietary fat has increased, so those who study food and nutrition have come to the conclusion that a high fat diet increases body weight. While it is true that a high fat diet can increase body weight, and American's have increased their fat intake over time, it is also important to point out that we have also increased our intake of refined fiber less foods and sugary foods at the same time. Plus, we expend less calories because the jobs of today require many to sit at a desk in front of a computer while many jobs in the past were more physical using more calories. I agree we are getting fatter as a nation due to a love for fattening foods, but I also believe many overlook the other facts. We are less active and we eat a poor choice of carbohydrate foods that are very refined and lack a high fiber content.

When dietary fat enters the body, it is used as fuel and any excess is efficiently stored in fat stores. Remember way back where I showed you how I need 1800 calories a day doing nothing, at rest. That means I need only 75 calories per hour (1800 calories divided by 24). Also, recall the body uses primarily fat as a fuel source at rest. Fat is a major fuel source and it is easy to overload the body with calories. When too much dietary fat and calories enters the body, the excess is stored.

When fat enters the body, it is broken down into its two raw components, fatty acids and glycerol. Fatty acids can fuel the muscles and glycerol can be "re-manufactured" into glucose. This glucose can be used by the blood, just like the glucose from carbohydrates and it can be used by the brain, as the brain relies on glucose as its fuel.

If the body does not need the fat as fuel it will put the fatty acids and glycerol back together and store the fat in body fat stores.

It is thought that carbohydrates, calorie for calorie, have a less tendency to be stored as fat than dietary fat. This is true because when carbohydrates are eaten in excess, they must make glycerol first. Glycerol combines with fatty acids to form fat. This "new fat" can be stored as body fat. Dietary fat already exists as dietary fat (three fatty acids and glycerol) which the body can readily store when excess calories are consumed. Carbs also exert a greater thermic effect than fat, leaving less calories available to the body. (see Chapter 11: THERMOGENESIS)

Saturated Fats: A Nemis To Muscle

There are different types of dietary fats. Saturated fats are solid at room temperature and unsaturated fats are liquid at room temperature. All animal sources of fat, like the fat found in meats, chicken, in eggs and dairy products (unless they are the fat free version) contain saturated fats. Saturated fats, consumed in excess, can exert a negative effect on the cardiovascular system. Saturated fats can clog the arteries, forcing the heart to work overtime to pump blood throughout the body. They also cause the blood to become thick and syrup-like, which makes it more difficult for the blood to reach the organs and tissues. From a body fat standpoint, saturated fats can damage the outer cell of muscle tissue, which indirectly may aggravate and enhance fat storage.

Insulin Insensitive Muscle Is Body Fat Friendly

Saturated fats can damage the outer portion of cells. Other potential damagers to the cell include

stress,	a high amount of body fat
alcohol,	a lack of exercise
smoking,	a low fiber intake
the use of drugs,	a high sugar diet
	a refined carbohydrate diet

All these factors can damage the cell's ability to use glucose. If the cell becomes resistant to using glucose as a fuel, the body adjusts and responds by trying to force the glucose in the blood into the muscle tissue. It does so, by releasing more insulin - the storage hormone that is required to "get" sugar into tissues.

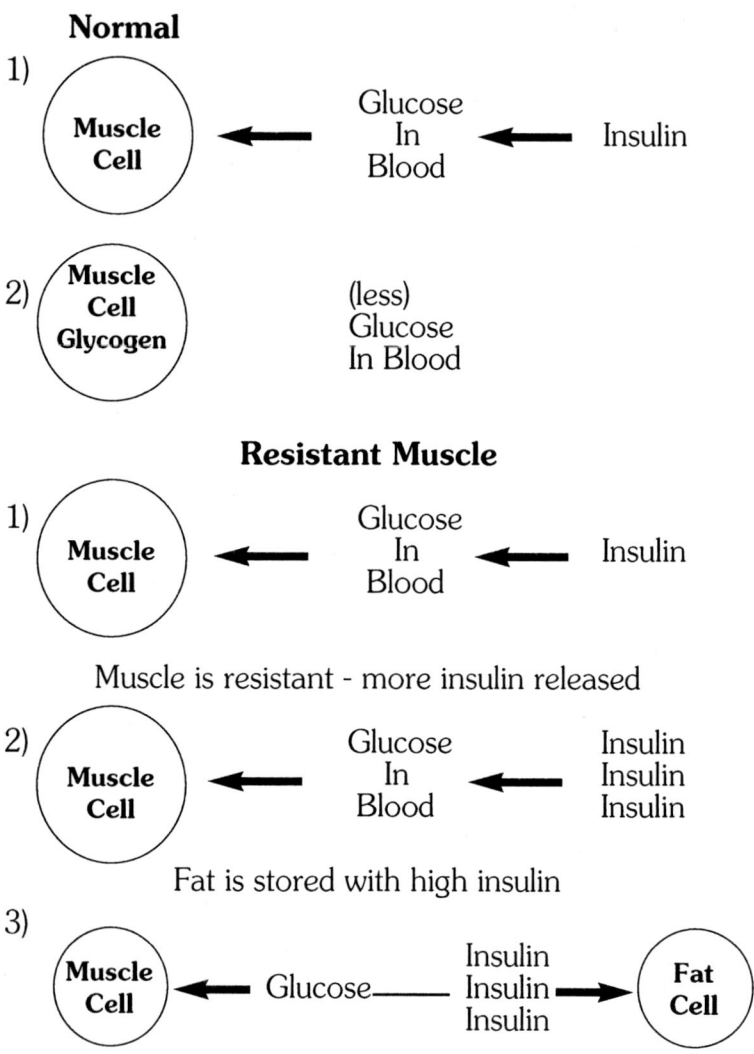

Normal

1) Muscle Cell ← Glucose In Blood ← Insulin

2) Muscle Cell Glycogen — (less) Glucose In Blood

Resistant Muscle

1) Muscle Cell ← Glucose In Blood ← Insulin

Muscle is resistant - more insulin released

2) Muscle Cell ← Glucose In Blood ← Insulin Insulin Insulin

Fat is stored with high insulin

3) Muscle Cell ← Glucose —— Insulin Insulin Insulin → Fat Cell

There are receptors for insulin on both muscle cells and fat cells. When a muscle cell is less sensitive to insulin (caused by the factors on page 33) the fat cell receptors become more sensitive. In an attempt to get glucose into the muscle cells, which are now stubborn and resistant to insulin, the body releases more insulin. Unfortunately high insulin tends to cause some of the glucose to be diverted towards the fat cells. When muscle cells become resistant to insulin, correspondingly, fat cells become more sensitive to insulin. The net effect is fat is more likely to be stored.

Muscle Reverses Insulin Resistance

Adding muscle via a solid weight training program coupled with a low sugar, low refined carbohydrate, high fiber diet is the fastest way to make muscles more sensitive to insulin.

When muscles become sensitive to insulin, the body releases less insulin.

This is like a seesaw effect (see chart).

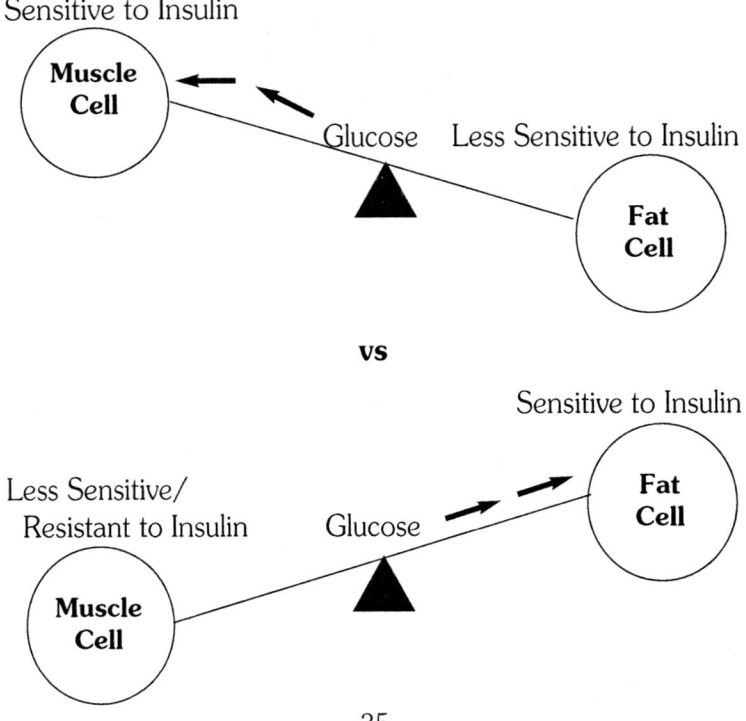

Sensitive to Insulin

Muscle Cell

Glucose   Less Sensitive to Insulin

Fat Cell

vs

Sensitive to Insulin

Less Sensitive/ Resistant to Insulin   Glucose

Fat Cell

Muscle Cell

Fiber, Fish, and Chromium

Besides having a lean body that is high in muscle, there are other ways to make muscle more sensitive to insulin. Remember, making the muscle more sensitive to insulin can lead to a leaner physique as high insulin levels, produced with insulin insensitivity, can lead to fat storage.

Chromium, a trace mineral, fish fat found in supplemental form as omega-3 fatty acids and found in fatty fish like salmon, mackerel, tuna, sardines, and herring and fiber found naturally in foods, especially in vegetables and oats, make a muscle more sensitive to insulin.

If a muscle is more sensitive to insulin, less net insulin has to be produced. Lower insulin will more likely store excess glucose in muscle and liver stores, unless those stores are already full. If muscle and liver stores are full, the body will store carbohydrates as fat.

Chapter Four

How Many Calories Do I Need?

So far, you can refer back to chapter 3 where I showed you the amount of calories I need in one day. Let's get more specific.

First, it is important to re-establish the lowest amount of calories a person needs in one day. This can be found by testing your body fat. A simple body fat test will tell you what percentage of your body is fat. A person who weighs 150 pounds and is 15% body fat has 22.5 pounds of fat and 128 pounds of muscle. Let's take a look:

Weight: 150 pounds

15% fat	
150	150 pounds
.15	- 22.5 pounds of fat
22.5 pounds of fat	127.5 pounds muscle/lean body mass

A person who contains 127 pounds of lean body mass will require 1270 (127 + 0) calories a day. This number is called your *Basal Metabolism (BM).* Basal metabolism is the number of calories you need in a day to maintain your muscle mass, to provide fuel for the organs, and brain. This is the minimum required to maintain life.

Many diets call for a caloric intake that is less than 1270 calories. Men, and especially women, who weigh less than 150 pounds will require less calories and have a lower basal metabolism while those who weigh more or those who carry more muscle will have a higher basal metabolism, and will require more calories.

Basal metabolism does not take into consideration the extra energy demands of digestion of foods nor the very real and high energy demands of everyday life and exercise.

Reducing calories below basal metabolism requirements, will cause the body to tap muscle and organs as fuel. It will lead to exhaustion, lethargy and the diet will be too restrictive to maintain for any length of time. This is the exact scenario of many who have failed time after time using diets that are just too low in caloric value. Fat is lost but muscle mass and energy are sacrificed.

Also, when calories remain below basal metabolism requirements for too long, the body will "make the low calorie level go like the previous higher calorie intake." I like this analogy. If you are earning $4000 a month but your boss suddenly cuts your pay to $2500 a month, you will try to live the same lifestyle on $2500 as you did on $4000 a month. After a while, you have to adjust and save money, and change your lifestyle. The same is true with a caloric intake that is simply too low. When calories are cut below basal metabolic needs, the body will accommodate and slow its metabolism, so it becomes difficult to lose fat even on low calories. The engine in your body, that basal metabolism, can adjust and burn at a lower level when calories are cut too low for too long.

What About The Calories I Need After Getting Out Of Bed

After establishing the lowest amount of calories a person can eat without the basal metabolism slowing, one must establish how many calories he needs to fit his specific lifestyle.

Therefore, calories must be added to the basal metabolism, so a person can perform chores, work, and exercise.

Here is an easy way to establish additional caloric needs.

Basal Metabolism (BM): 1270 calories

Next, add to the BM more calories based on your lifestyle.

For The Extremely Active	:	BM x 1 + BM
For Very Active	:	BM x .7 + BM
For Moderately Active	:	BM x .4 + BM
For Non Active	:	BM x .2 + BM

Therefore a person who is extremely active and has a basal metabolism of 127 (because he has 127 pounds of muscle) will need 2540 calories in a day. An active, moderately active, and non active person with a BM of 127 will need 2159 calories, 1778 calories, and 1524 calories respectively.

The definitions are:

Extremely Active: Work a physical job, construction, mail carrier, builder, landscaper, AND work out hard 6 or more times a week.

Very Active: Either work a physical job and exercise hard 3 times a week, OR a desk job and work out hard 6 times a week.

Moderately Active: Desk job and work out 4 to 5 times a week OR a physical job and do not exercise.

Non Active: Neither exercise nor work a physical job.

Adding muscle mass is really the most effective, efficient, long range, successful way to lose body fat. Muscle increases the basal metabolism. If the person with 127 pounds of muscle mass begins a weight training program and adds ten pounds of muscle mass in one year, she will now have 137 pounds of lean muscle mass, and require 1370 (137 + 0 = 1370) calories a day, at rest.

Adding muscle increases Basal Metabolism!

What About Carbohydrates, Protein and Fat?

Once you choose the calorie level that is best suited for you, you will need to find requirements for protein, carbohydrates, and fat.

Finding the amount of fat you need is easy. Just avoid *extra* fat found in butter and salad dressings, avoid sauces, avoid fattier cuts of meat, and watch out for sauteed vegetables and restaurant meals that are often high in fat. Fat is often hidden. You ask the waitress if an item on the menu is made with butter, oil, or margarine, and she replies, "hardly any at all-just a tad to flavor the food." Well, that tad is more likely a ton, which adds a lot of fat and a lot of calories.

My advice is to eat a very low fat diet. This will still provide you with more fat than you think. All foods have fat, some in tiny amounts, and there is fat in fish and chicken. Trying to eat a very low fat diet usually will come out to a diet that yields 10 to 15% fat.

Let's look at our example of the woman who has 137 pounds of lean body mass and a BM of 1370 calories and is *Moderately Active*. She is consuming 1524 calories a day.

Ten to 15% of those calories will contain fat even on a "low fat" diet. Here is the math:

$$\begin{array}{ll} 1524 & \text{Calories a Day} \\ \underline{\times\ .15} & \\ 228 & \text{Calories of Fat} \end{array}$$

These fat calories, are mostly found in the protein foods one consumes: chicken breast, turkey breast, lean cuts of beef and fish. Whole grain breads, brown rice, pasta and potatoes also contain small amounts of dietary fat.

The goal is to find how much protein and carbohydrates to eat. The next step is to subtract the fat calories from the total calories.

> 1524 total calories
> - 228 fat calories
> 1296 calories remaining

Find The Protein

Protein needs are correlated with lean body mass. The more muscle one carries, the more protein is needed.

Bodybuilders, the leanest athletes on the face of the earth, usually consume at least one gram of protein for every pound of lean body mass.

In our example, the female has 137 pounds of lean body mass. If you are training with weights to increase your basal metabolism, you should follow their advice and eat more protein. One gram of protein yields four calories.

Protein, unlike fat or carbohydrates, can not be stored to any significant degree. Therefore, it is important to eat protein at each meal.

At 4 meals, the breakdown looks like this:

Meal 1	34 grams of protein
Meal 2	34 grams of protein
Meal 3	34 grams of protein
Meal 4	34 grams of protein

Each gram of protein yields four calories. So, 137 grams multiplied by 4 = 548 calories of protein.

Applied to the example we have been using:

$$
\begin{array}{rl}
1296 & \text{calories remaining} \\
- 548 & \text{calories of protein} \\
\hline
748 & \text{calories remaining}
\end{array}
$$

Finding Carbohydrates

The last macronutrient to find is carbohydrates. Like protein, carbohydrates yield 4 calories a gram.

748 calories/4 = 187 grams of carbohydrates

In the example we have been using, the person is eating four meals a day. Therefore, 44 grams of carbohydrates can be eaten at each meal.

Meal 1	34 grams protein	44 grams carbohydrates
Meal 2	34 grams protein	44 grams carbohydrates
Meal 3	34 grams protein	44 grams carbohydrates
Meal 4	34 grams protein	44 grams carbohydrates
	137 grams protein	187 grams carbohydrates

Sample Diets Yielding Approximately 187 Grams Carbohydrates 137 Grams Protein

MEAL 1
7 egg whites
1 slice fat free cheese
T. fat free cream cheese
1 bagel

MEAL 2
7 oz. chicken breast (PCW)
small salad w/ fat free dressing
6 oz. potato (PCW)

MEAL 3
1 cup rice
1/3 cup beans
5 oz. ground round steak (PCW)

MEAL 4
1 tuna burger (see Appendage 1))
2 slices whole grain bread
lettuce, tomatoes, mustard,
fat free mayonnaise

PCW= "pre cooked weight"

MEAL 1
5 egg whites
1 egg
1/2 banana
2 oz. oatmeal (PCW)

MEAL 2
4 oz. sliced turkey
2 slices fat free cheese
salad w/ 2 oz. pasta
    (PCW)
2 T. Laura's dressing
    (see Appendage 1)

MEAL 3
7 large shrimp
2 oz. pasta (PCW)
cup vegetables w/ low fat
    dressing

MEAL 4
7 oz. white fish
cup vegetables
2 servings no fat french
fries   (see Appendage 1)

Review Questions

Q: I want to lose weight as fast as possible, how much weight can I expect to lose a week?

A: It is realistic to lose 1 to 3 pounds of weight each week. If you are trying to lose 10 to 15 pounds, shoot for 1 pound a week. If you are trying to lose 16 to 30 pounds, look for 2 pounds of weight loss each week. Finally, if you have a lot of fat to lose, more than 30 pounds, it is ok to lose 3 pounds a week.

Q: What if I lose more than the prescribed weekly amount?

A: If you are losing more than the prescribed amount, you are losing more than fat. When too much weight is shed, the body will start to burn muscle tissue. Remember, muscle increases basal metabolism (BM). Losing muscle will decrease the BM, making fat loss more difficult because of a slower BM.

Q: Can I lose weight without exercising?

A: Absolutely. If you plan your diet carefully, it is possible to shed fat and weight without exercise. People GAIN weight by food alone. An excess calorie intake will stimulate fat storage, so a decrease in caloric intake will cause fat breakdown.

Maximizing Fat Loss With Diet

Once establishing calorie requirements, protein requirements, carbohydrate requirements and fat requirements (found naturally in a low fat diet) the dietary goal is to alter the diet as much as possible to allow for maximal fat loss without a loss in energy. Many mistakenly cut calories too low to maximize fat loss, but run into a roadblock. Reducing calories too quickly or too low will cause the BM to decrease due to a loss in muscle mass. And more importantly,

> while the job of fat cells is to expand in size on a calorically excessive diet, fat cells will hold onto, hoard, and resist breakdown when calories are too low.

There is a smarter way to maximize fat loss. It is possible to maximize fat loss through exercise and by *inhibiting* fat storage.

Muscle Burns Fat!!

Adding muscle mass will increase BM so more calories are required at rest.

Fat Inhibition

One of the biggest mistakes many dieters make is to conceptualize weight loss, or to think of losing fat in these terms: restriction, reduction, starving, cutting, and calorie deprivation.

Calorie restriction definitely works. But the restriction, or the cut in calories, ought to be a very small amount. Many will quickly cut calories from a very high amount to a low amount. When calories are cut too severely, the fat cells can hoard fat. Reductions should be made very slowly. With small cuts in calories, the body will recognize the deficit, and start to allow fat to be tapped to be used as fuel. The deficit should be 10 to 15% to start. A person eating 2000 calories a day can reduce by 10% or 200 calories or by 15% 300 calories to 1800 or 1700 respectively. This small cut will set fat burning in motion without setting off an emergency starvation alarm in the fat cells which would cause the fat cells to fight back by hoarding fat. A small cut will also allow you to stay energetic so you can continue to have fuel to continue with your day to day life. Fat loss can only be coaxed, not forced!

A better approach to fat loss is to eat enough calories to fuel your BM and to accommodate your activity level (see page 39). Next, avoid foods that cause high insulin release, and break your meals into small more frequent meals.

A person who eats 1524 calories a day in one meal will store plenty of that intake as body fat. The body will take what it needs at the one meal and store the rest. Some will enter muscle glycogen stores, while the majority will be stored as body fat. The more meals, the better as 1524 calories divided into 5 or 6 meals will have a less likely chance to be stored as body fat. When fat is **not** lost, but is prevented from being stored, as with a 5 to 6 meal plan, a low sugar diet, and a moderate calorie diet, *Fat Inhibition* is occurring. If I gave you a pill to inhibit fat from being stored on your body for the rest of your life, all you would need to do is burn off the fat you are carrying, and you would achieve your "dream body." In most bodies, fat is always being stored, to a small degree, and burned off, to a small degree. You want to set up your diet to inhibit the storage and initiate fat burning with a very small cut in calories and by splitting your total calorie intake into 5 to 6 meals. I discussed insulin

47

release and its effects on fat storage. Eating 5 to 6 meals, within your caloric needs, will force you to control insulin levels by controlling how many carbohydrates are consumed at each meal.

Let's divide the previous meal plan of 1524 calories and 137 grams of protein and 187 grams of carbohydrates into 6 meals. The new breakdown would look like this:

Meal 1   23 grams protein   31 grams carbohydrates
Meal 2   23 grams protein   31 grams carbohydrates
Meal 3   23 grams protein   31 grams carbohydrates
Meal 4   23 grams protein   31 grams carbohydrates
Meal 5   23 grams protein   31 grams carbohydrates
Meal 6   23 grams protein   31 grams carbohydrates

Sample Diet Yielding Approximately
187 Grams Carbohydrates • 137 Grams Protein

MEAL 1
4 egg whites
slice fat free cheese
1 1/2 oz. oatmeal (or) 1 english muffin

MEAL 2
4 oz. chicken breast (PCW)
1 1/2 oz. pasta (PCW) mixed w/ a small salad
fat free and low sugar dressing

MEAL 3
3/4 cup non fat cottage cheese mixed w/
1 cup cooked rice
add cinnamon and EQUAL

MEAL 4
3 oz. lean roast beef
1 slice fat free cheese
1 pita pocket
lettuce, tomato, onion, fat free mayo, mustard

MEAL 5
2 cups no-sugar and fat free vanilla yogurt

MEAL 6
6 oz. scallops (PCW)
salad
5 oz. potato

PCW= "pre cooked weight"

Review Questions

Q: What is the purpose of eating smaller meals?

A: Smaller meals break your carbohydrate intake into smaller, but more frequent portions. Carbs are the double edge sword in weight loss. They provide fuel, yet in excess, or when there is too much sugar from carbs in the blood at one time, fat can be stored, and fat breakdown ceases.

Q: Are there other benefits of smaller meals?

A: Yes, smaller meals allow for better nutrient absorption.

Q: If I eat the right number of calories for the amount of lean body mass I carry and eat six meals a day, isn't it impossible to gain fat?

A: Well, it becomes more difficult. But, if you eat poor sources of carbohydrates, ones that lack fiber, like simple carbohydrates, and if you do not eat vegetables that contain plenty of fiber, it is still possible, to not lose fat. But, if you eat the right types of carbohydrates, it would be very likely that you would lose body fat.

Chapter Five

The Role of Exercise On Fat Loss

Fat can be lost by eating the right diet, one that matches your BM and activity level. Your diet must inhibit fat from being stored by eating several smaller meals comprised of natural carbohydrates, high fiber and avoiding sugar and simple carbohydrates.

Many believe that exercise is the only way to lose fat. I disagree. While it is definitely helpful, the way we eat is more important in controlling body fat.

Diet exerts a tremendous influence on general health. A poor diet is correlated with some forms of diabetes and heart disease including strokes and heart attacks. Cancers can grow at a faster rate with a poor diet. Colon cancer, stomach cancer, breast cancer, prostate cancer and many others are associated with a poor diet. The wrong diet will make you fat and the best diet will make you lean. Yes, it is possible to achieve a low level of body fat with diet alone!

However, an overwhelming amount of evidence has shown that exercise combined with the right diet can lead to either faster fat loss or more permanent fat loss. On the other hand it is possible to exercise religiously, but eat a bad diet, and not lose fat! The wrong diet can turn on fat storage to the point where heavy exercise may not be able to override the body's constant attempt to store fat. The wrong diet can inhibit **all** fat breakdown exercise imparts!

There are two types of exercise: aerobic exercise and anaerobic exercise. One is only moderately helpful in achieving a low level of body fat while the other is the absolute key in achieving a fit, trim (and muscular) body.

Aerobic exercise, running, cycling, stair climbing, and rowing, can burn calories, but the burning torch that aerobics ignite can soon cool to nothing greater than a flickering flame. I'll explain.

Aerobics burns calories. High intensity aerobic exercise burns about 10 calories a minute. An untrained person, desiring to shed fat, who walks on an inclined treadmill for one hour will burn approximately 600 calories.

Nutritionists agree a pound of fat will be shed from the body when a person expends 3500 calories. If the person who exercised aerobically for an hour and burned 600 calories repeats this 6 days a week, he will have burned off a total of 3600 calories, about a pound of fat.

If the same person continues to exercise, 6 days a week, each and every week, for a full year, we would expect a weight loss of 52 pounds. However, the reality is a loss of about half that amount.

Here in lies the reason. The body adapts to aerobic

exercise by becoming efficient. By the fourth week into the training sessions, the body begins to adapt and performs the same amount of physical work, by expending or burning less calories. By the 52nd week, the body can walk the treadmill at the same incline and burn as few as 300 calories an hour.

This adaptation phenomena is also seen in dieting. A person who is eating 3000 calories a day, but reduces his caloric intake to 2500 a day will create a deficit of 500 a day. This should account for 3500 calories a week or one pound of fat.

However, one year into the diet of 2500 calories, the body definitely will not have shed 52 pounds of fat. The body adapts to caloric reduction by eventually slowing its overall metabolism, or by making the "most" out of the 2500 calorie intake.

The only way to change your body, the only way to lose fat and keep it off for good, and the only way to alter your metabolism and to create a better one is with regular weight training coupled with a diet that provides enough calories to match your BM and your level of activity.

Weight training is very different from aerobic training. With aerobic training, calories are burned. However, the adaptation process causes the body to burn less calories with the exercise over time. With weight training, there is a very different and unique adaptation process. That adaptation is an increase in muscle mass.

Increasing muscle mass increases basal metabolism (BM), the amount of calories you need at complete rest. A person who weights 127 and needs 1270 calories a day at complete rest (see Chapter 3) will need more calories with an increase in muscle mass (lean body mass). Adding 10 pounds of muscle, which for most people would require 6 to 12 months of supervised weight training will elevate the metabolism by 100 calories a day. Now the lean body mass is 137 and the person will need 1370 calories at complete rest.

An increase in body mass of 10 pounds, creating a need for another 100 calories daily, is a simple way to increase your metabolism. Dieting can decrease metabolism while adding muscle can increase it, regardless of changes in eating habits.

So far, it looks like this

127 pounds LBM	137 pounds LBM
▼	▼
1270 calories required	1370 calories required

With no change in eating habits (no increase or decrease in caloric consumption) and a 100 calorie deficit a day produced by the addition of 10 pounds of lean body mass will automatically use up 700 calories a week.

If 3500 calories is equal to one pound of fat, it will take 35 days to burn off one pound of fat, *"Without Trying."* Therefore, about ten pounds of fat will be lost in one year, as a result of increasing lean body mass by 10 pounds.

Three More Ways To Lose Fat By Adding Ten Pounds of LBM

1) The ten pounds of fat lost in one year as a result of adding 10 pounds of lean body mass, does not take into consideration the effort required (i.e. the calories burned off) in trying to build the ten pounds of muscle. Training with weights requires energy. If there is no great increase in calories while training to gain the ten pounds, much of the calories burned off will come from body fat, while some calories will come from the foods eaten. If the foods consumed are used training with weights, then there will be less net calories left over to be stored as fat. Training to build muscle burns calories from foods and fat stores leading to fat loss.

2) Recovery requires calories. When you train with weights, the stress placed upon the muscles actually causes micro tears or micro damage to the muscles that are worked. In order to grow or to add new muscle, the body must repair the damaged muscles. Once damaged muscles are repaired, they become ever so slightly denser and larger. The recovery/repair process requires additional calories! When a person does aerobics, there is no significant trauma to the muscles. But a person who lifts weights will tear down muscle tissue and RESTING muscles need extra fuel to repair the muscular damage brought on by weight training.

3) Adding muscle changes the metabolism of sugar. Recall there are receptors for insulin on both fat cells and muscle cells. They act in a see-saw like fashion. If one is sensitive to the effects of insulin, the other is

correspondingly insensitive. Adding muscle makes muscle cells more sensitive to insulin which means the fat cells become slightly less sensitive to insulin. This is important because insulin sensitive muscles do not require a large insulin output. High insulin levels tend to store some carbohydrates as fat while lower insulin levels will more likely shuttle carbohydrates towards muscle.

Case Study: Susan Richards

Susan Richards came to my fitness weekend a few years ago. She was 42 years old, 40 pounds overweight, yet a compulsive aerobic athlete. She had been running about 20 miles a week, on average, for 5 years. She came to my camp totally discouraged. She couldn't lose weight even though she averaged 20 miles a week worth of running. Admittedly, her diet was not the greatest, but, she reasoned, "Shouldn't the running be burning something?"

I explained to her the phenomena that I explained in this chapter: how the body adapts to cardiovascular exercise. It gets better at doing it, and it tries to expend as few calories as possible because the body is trying to run longer and longer, further and further. I went on to ask her who she thought was leaner, the female sprinters at the Olympics or the Marathoners? We agreed the sprinters looked incredibly lean, seemingly devoid of fat, while the Marathoners appeared thin, yet soft. Their legs and arms jiggle when they run, while the sprinters, whose event is definitely anaerobic, stop and go and similar to bodybuilding training, are awesomely lean and hard looking.

So far so good, but Susan's greatest fear was to quit running. Again, she reasoned, "If I quit won't I gain a ton of weight because I will be expending less?" While I appreciated her reasoning, I had to disagree, offering the advice that her metabolism could be slow due to the "aerobic adaptation response." Furthermore, we concluded, after a thorough examination of her diet records, she would often overeat thinking she needed the energy to complete her run!

After much haggling, I helped her develop a four day a week training session, with weights and no cardio work. She also adjusted her diet to utilize some sound nutrition principles. After a 7 month period, Susan lost 14 pounds on the scale and had to revamp her wardrobe because her clothes became so loose fitting. We never did take her body fat, because she was too self conscientious, so I do not know how much total fat she lost. Essentially, she lost a lot of fat without performing any cardio work, whereas she never lost fat before performing 20 plus miles of hard aerobic work a week.

Chapter Six

Varying Caloric Intake:
Metabolic Trickery

Many people, who claim, not to be big eaters, often store a lot of body fat without eating an excessive amount of calories. Remember the example where it is possible to exercise every day and not achieve the fat loss you desire nor lose the amount of fat you expect because the body adapts to aerobic exercise by becoming metabolically efficient?

Well, many have a tougher time shedding fat and are effective fat storers due to a sporadic, unplanned, and inconsistent diet. Most people eat a wide variation of total calories each day. At my weekend fitness retreats, I have clients keep a 3, 5, or 7 day food log. I ask each person to record each day the exact foods and the exact quantities of food they eat. Then, I simply help them tally up the calories for each day. Here is an example of a sporadic calorie intake. Notice how it varies greatly from day to day.

Day 1	2300 calories	(Monday)
Day 2	1400 calories	(Tuesday)
Day 3	2000 calories	(Wednesday)
Day 4	2600 calories	(Thursday)
Day 5	1900 calories	(Friday)
Day 6	3400 calories	(Saturday)
Day 7	1200 calories	(Sunday)

On a graph, this looks like this:

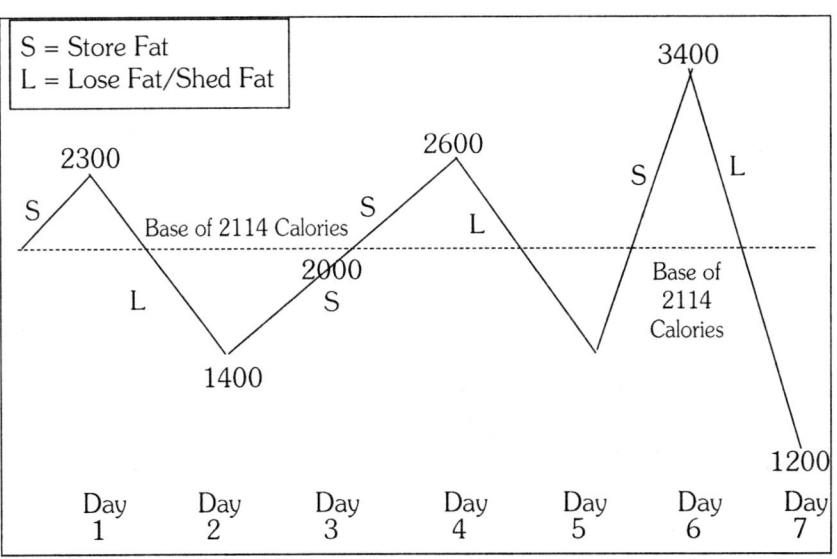

Here is the problem, "metabolic confusion" really, that can lead to fat storage.

On Monday, the person starts the week with 2300 calories and cuts back to 1400 on Tuesday. With this reduction, the body reacts by giving up some fat as fuel. After all, 1400 is less than 2300 and a caloric deficit is required to initiate fat burning.

On Wednesday, she consumed 2000 calories. Two things will happen. Either the body will perceive 2000 as

300 calories less than 2300 so fat may be given up as fuel, or it may not allow fat to be released to be used up as fuel because Wednesday's intake of 2000 is higher than Tuesday's 1400 calorie intake.

Thursday, she eats 2600 which is definitely higher than both Tuesday and Wednesday, so the body is in a fat storing mode on Thursday.

Friday, she finds herself busy at work getting ready for a hectic weekend, and she could not find time in the day to eat as much as usual. At 1900 calories, she should tap some fat as fuel as Friday's caloric intake is lower than the previous days intake.

Saturday includes splurging on lunch and desert at the mall and her husband takes her out for dinner later in the evening. At dinner she indulges as many who dine out, myself included, are apt to do. Saturday's tally comes in at 3400 calories, definitely enough to store fat and, since the body will correctly perceive that the 3400 intake is higher than all the other days, it will turn fat storage on, probably into high gear.

Sunday morning she wakes up early knowing she ate too much the night before. Wanting to "make up" or "correct" the damage incurred on Saturday, she cuts way back on Sunday, hoping to jump start fat breakdown, and to get an early start on her new diet, to start the following day.

The best step, to correct such sporadic eating habits which send conflicting and confusing messages to the body and can lead to fat storage, regardless of caloric intake, is to take the average of the seven day food intake, and start anew.

If you add up all the calories that were consumed in

the week, the total is 14,798. Dividing 14,798 by 7, yields an average of 2114 calories a day. Eating the same amount of calories, particularly in the same amount of meals, 5 or 6 meals being optimal, will prevent conflicting signals to fat metabolism. When the same person commits to eating a sound, steady and regular meal plan of 4 to 6 meals of the same amount of calories each and every day, the body will be able to respond in a more sane and regular fashion so fat storage is not always being stimulated. Irregular eating and irregular caloric intakes should be avoided for those seeking optimal energy and lower body fat levels.

The eating patterns above is a reason many who reduce calories never seem to lose fat. If the person who eats such a varying diet cuts her calories down, say to 1600 calories a day, the body will not immediately be able to give up fat as fuel because it will not readily recognize the deficit. Her body is used to deficits. In the example, she created deficits from the mean of 2114 calories on four different days, but she was above this level on 3 days. Every time a caloric deficit was created, it was broken with an increase in calories. Her body has become conditioned. Her body is thinking, "When calories are reduced do not give up fat as fuel because the deficit will soon cease, and I will get more than enough calories to survive and store for the next deficit!"

The only way her body will ever be able to recognize a deficit is to create a base, 2114 calories and eat that amount day in and day out, for a period of 2 to 3 months. After 3 months of eating the same amount of calories each day, her body will recognize and respond to a deficit by giving up fat as fuel.

Making A Deficit or Adding Exercise

Once a **Base** diet is established, in this case, approximately 2100 calories, and the base is followed consistently for at least four months, you can induce a calorie deficit to cause the body to call upon fat stores for energy. Establishing the base will allow your body to respond to the deficit while sporadic eating will inhibit the body from responding to any dietary manipulations.

As I noted earlier, the body will react to small changes in caloric intake. Large and sudden caloric reductions will temporarily work, but the body will quickly fight back by trying to hoard fat.

To lose body fat and to avoid a metabolic slowdown that is associated with severe calorie reductions, try cutting calories by 10 to 15% maximum. The body will recognize and react to a smaller deficit by giving up fat as fuel. Many believe they can lose fat by making severe cuts. They hope that cutting way back on calories will force the body to shed fat. Cutting way back will work for about five or six days, then the body will lower its metabolic rate to protect itself from whittling away to nothing. Finally, the diet and reduction will take its toll on the dieter. It will not provide enough calories to think clear or to do any type of physical work. Hunger pains will eventually override those with the strongest willpower. The end result of a severe cut in calories will be a slower metabolism, fading weight loss, a loss of energy, and extreme hunger. In total, this will lead to breaking the diet by eating all the forbidden foods that will now be more readily stored as fat due to the metabolic slowdown that accompanies a severe reduction in calories.

After establishing a base diet, the other option is to add exercise, specifically weight training exercises. Eating the same caloric intake, while increasing muscle mass through weight training burns calories, some coming from fat stores, and it increases lean body mass which will increase the metabolism. A faster metabolism is one of the secrets to long range and permanent weight loss.

I don't think cutting calories while increasing activity is a good idea. Changing more than one variable at a time can mislead you. If a person established a base diet, and reduced calories by 10 to 15%, and lost fat, but has recently reached a sticking point, he should do one of three things. Reduce calories, or manipulate caloric intake or increase the amount of calories he expends through exercise. Cutting calories a bit lower may work, but it could also lead to a slight slowdown in the metabolic rate. Performing aerobic work will help, but it could also lead to an adaptation down the road where the body adapts to the aerobic activity by expending less calories doing the same amount of work. Adding weight training, or embarking on a *serious* weight training schedule will add more muscle to the body which will, in turn, beef up the metabolism.

Many who start a diet program AND an exercise program at the same time will also reach plateaus. For them, the solution to overcoming the plateau is sometimes confusing. The person knows his program was working but is perplexed as to which variable he should change to continue his weight loss. Should he exercise more? Or, should he cut calories? Was the diet more responsible for his physical changes or was the exercise the stimulus that caused the changes. Confused, but enthused, he changes both, and cuts calories and increases his activity. While this may work to overcome the dreaded plateau, it could lead to fatigue because its hard to exercise more while supplying the body with less fuel. Also, a combination of an increase in expenditure with a decrease in calories could lead to a **Perceived Large Deficit**. Remember, when calories are cut too low, the body starts to resist fat loss. Only subtle changes are required to overcome plateaus.

Varying Intake: **When It's Permissible**

Previously, I showed you why a diet that is sporadic or lacks consistency can send conflicting messages to the body regarding fat loss or fat storage. Without a base, the body doesn't really know what to respond to. When calories are higher for a day the body is good at storing fat and when calories are lower, the body may not allow fat cells to be broken down.

However, a variable caloric intake *after a base has been established, can lead to continual fat loss without a reduction in calories.* Let's say in the example we have been using, the person has been eating 2100 calories for an extended period of time. To lose fat she never cut calories, but added weight training, three times a week. Without cutting calories, she has lost fat by expending fuel and by adding muscle. More muscle has increased her metabolism, so she burns more fuel in a day, even while sitting in her office from 9 to 5 at work. Remember, recovery in weight training is very special and very different from recovery in aerobic exercise. To recover with from weight training means the body has to "repair" and "rebuild" muscle tissue that is broken down during weight training sessions. This special recovery requires calories (fuel). Since the person we are dealing with never added or cut calories from her diet, some of the fuel for recovery must come from fat stores!

So far, so good. However, with time, she is seeing less changes in her body and she wants to overcome a sticking point in her fat loss. She could increase her workouts, but she feels she is already working as hard as possible. An option is to vary her caloric intake. Remember, her base was established by finding her daily average caloric intake by adding up all the calories she ate in a week and dividing by 7. After eating 2100 calories a day, she has seemed to reach a sticking point. The body can be temporarily tricked into breaking down fat by reducing calories for three days and increasing them for one day. Here is how it works.

Recall from Chapter 3, I explained that excess carbohydrate intake can be stored in three places: muscle, liver, and fat. At 2100 calories, the woman has lost fat and increased muscle. She has not gained fat, so we know that her muscle reserves for carbohydrates are rarely full. When muscle stores of carbohydrates are full, the body will store the carbohydrates as body fat. If she has reached a plateau, perhaps, through adaptation, the carbohydrates that she is eating are now enough to saturate up her muscle stores so some of the calories from carbohydrates are preventing fat breakdown. This is just my theory, because the tips I am going to show

65

you below work, but no one really knows for sure exactly how they work.

Here are the carbohydrates, protein and fat the woman should be eating based upon the guidelines found in Chapter 4. Assuming she weights, after a year of weight training, 152 pounds with 137 pounds of muscle and eats 2100 calories a day, she should eat 309 grams of carbohydrates, 137 grams of protein, and 15% of her calories (315 calories) will naturally come from fat. It may take 309 grams of carbohydrates a day to keep her muscle glycogen stores full. Cutting *carbohydrates* by 15% for three days will lower blood sugar levels, it will lower insulin levels, and it will stimulate the release of hormone sensitive lipase which will initiate fat burning. Furthermore, when muscle glycogen stores are lower fat is broken down to be used as fuel. Fifteen percent of 309 carbohydrates is 46 grams of carbohydrates. To stimulate fat burning, she can cut her carbs to 263 grams a day. (309 - 46 = 263)

We want continual fat loss without reducing calories, since calorie reduction can lead to a metabolic adaptation that triggers fat cells to hoard fat. Therefore, she can eat 263 grams of carbs a day (which is NOT 15% less calories) followed by one day back to 309 carbohydrates which brings her back to 2100 calories. Then she can go higher in carbs by 15% for one day to 330, and then repeat the full process. Overall her carb intake looks like this:

Normal: 309 grams a day
Day One, Two, Three at 263
Day Four: 309
Day Five: 330

Repeat

Normal: glycogen are full at 309 gms

1)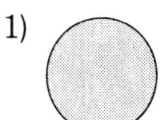

2) 263 carbs lower glycogen, stimulate fat breakdown
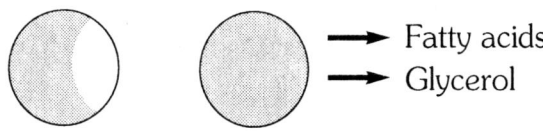

3) 309 carbs for one day
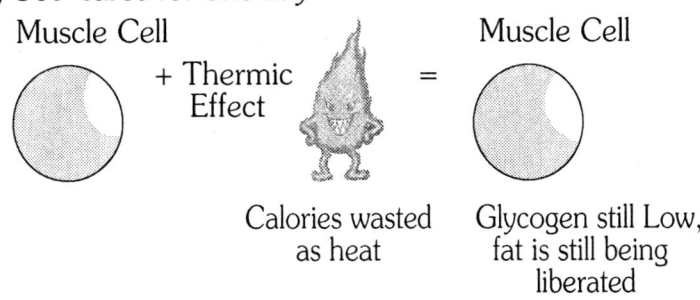

4) 330 carbs
Muscle Cell
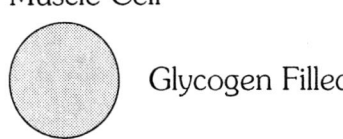

Glycogen Filled

After three days of lower carbs, the glycogen stores in the muscles become low. When carbs are reintroduced into a body that is "running low in muscle glycogen" the carbs will fill the muscle glycogen stores without being stored as fat. Glycogen hungry muscles take precedent (to store sugar from carbohydrates) over fat storage. Furthermore, carbohydrates have an interesting metabolic effect. Carbohydrates, cause an increase in metabolism. They do so by generating heat. Excess carbohydrates increase heat production and calorie burning when muscle glycogen stores are full.

Here, fat is broken down on days 1, 2, and 3 and excess carbohydrates exert a heat producing effect on day 4. Because of this effect, some of the carbohydrates have no real effect. The actual number is 309 grams a day, but due to an increase in heat, some are burned off as heat, leaving the net carbohydrate count lower, probably closer to 275 grams (see Chapter 11). This one day of a higher carb intake will not be sufficient to fill the glycogen stores back to normal, so fat burning continues. On day 5, the dieter increases carbohydrates high than normal to 330 grams a day. Some will be burned off as heat, but this should full glycogen stores back to normal. Then, the entire process is continued.

An interesting note. Notice *carbohydrate* intake was curtailed by 15%, *not calorie intake.*

Fifteen percent less calories would be 315 calories (2100 x .15 = 315)

But 15% less carbohydrates is only 185 calories! (309 x .15 = 46 grams of carbohydrates. One gram of carbohydrates = 4 calories. 46 x 4 = 185)

Therefore, fat loss is stimulated with a very minute

reduction in calories! We cut total carbohydrate calories by 15%, **not total calories!** Plus, we added more calories in for a day, without storing fat. Many people enjoy this type of diet because it allows them to have a day that is a bit higher in calories. The less we cut calories, the better!

While the type of variable dieting above, also known as rotational dieting, can lead to continual fat loss without any real significant reduction in calories, it should never be used by those who have not first established a base diet. A base diet is very important in establishing "regularity" to the metabolism so it is able to respond to small reductions in caloric intake.

Chapter Seven

The Weight Loss Accountant

So far we have been dealing with a lot of figures and calculations: total calories, calories from fat, calories from protein, calories from carbohydrates, grams of protein, grams of carbohydrates, percentages, etc. Surely, you will need a calculator to keep track of the many numbers which may have overwhelmed you by now.

Unfortunately, I feel number crunching is a very important part of learning about nutrition. You will never be able to build an exact diet, one that really works, and one that is built especially for you without knowing how to count calories, carbohydrates, protein, and fat. Starving doesn't really work for weight loss. The body simply slows its metabolism so fat loss becomes difficult and much of the weight loss comes from the burning of lean body mass. Eating a low fat diet can also be futile. I know many people who eat very little fat but are still carrying a lot of extra weight around. Calorie counting by itself could work but most end up losing weight, only to gain it right back. Exercise works, but a person must pay careful attention to total caloric intake, so more calories are expended than consumed. The best way to find out what you are eating, how much you are eating, (and the reason why you may not be shedding fat) is to write down and record all the foods you eat each and every day. Writing down the foods you eat will provide you with all the information you need to start a sound diet and eating program. Otherwise, if you do not know exactly how much and what you are eating, your diet is nothing more than a big guessing game. Will 1800 calories work? How would you know if you are not exactly sure how many calories you are eating? And if you start to lose fat on 1800 calories, is it too low in calories, or is the cut too severe which can lead to a road block down the fat loss road?

Unfortunately, when one starts to record the foods he eats, a strange phenomena occurs. People fudge. They alter eating habits. They eat better. They eat less. They eat low fat. They eat the right things and avoid the fattening things. So, food records are a must to start a program, but many should keep them for a couple of weeks, as it may take this time to finally find the "real way" you eat.

Many people resist the idea of keeping records of total calorie, carbohydrate, protein, and fat intake but are well aware they can not organize, control, and take charge of their financial lives without balancing a budget. A dietary budget will allow you to establish a starting point. It will show you the reason you are fatter than you want to be. When you start seeing progress, you will know why, and if your progress wanes, you have the information and numbers you will need to change to continue your progress.

What To Record

Here is what your records should show.
1) Time of day with the foods eaten: calories, carbohydrates, protein, and fat
2) Total calories for the day
3) Totals for carbohydrates, protein, and fat for the day
   ** See appendage 2 for food values.

71

Chapter Eight

Does 3500 Calories Equal One Pound of Fat?

There was a time when dieters counted only calories with little regard to fat intake, carbohydrate intake, individuality in metabolisms, etc. It was simple. Just count calories, cut a certain amount from the diet and fat loss will follow. Dieters who have failed over and over will realize there may be more to losing weight than simply counting calories.

Food scientists tell us one pound of fat can be shed when a total of 3500 calories is omitted form the diet. This is not exactly true. Let's look at an example.

A) John eats 3300 calories a day.
B) Jane eats 1800 calories a day.
    Both reduce their caloric intake by 500 daily creating a weekly deficit of 3500 calories respectively.
A) John now eats 2800 calories a day.
B) Jane now eats 1300 calories a day.

A) John reduces his calories by 500 a day, 3500 a week, or by 15%.
B) Jane reduces her calories by 500 a day, 3500 a week, or by 28%.

Using the popular premise that 3500 calories will equal one pound of fat, the two will actually see very different results. John can expect to lose one pound of fat a week because he has reduced his calories and is creating a one week deficit of 3500 calories. Furthermore, he can expect to continue to lose fat at a clip of a pound a week because the body will recognize the deficit and the deficit is only a 15% (mild) reduction.

Jane may not be as fortunate. She will also lose a pound of fat a week because she created a 3500 calorie deficit, but in doing so, she has cut her calories back too far, by 28%. Such a cut will eventually cause the body to start to fight back and resist fat loss as (in general) caloric reductions of greater than 15% will lead to muscle loss which will slow down the metabolism, making fat loss slower. Jane COULD continue to lose a pound of weight each week, but much will come from muscle and a loss of muscle will slow the metabolism.

For fat loss, aim for a reduction in calories as a percentage of your base. Reducing by 15% will lead to fat loss without slowing down the metabolism because muscle is more likely to be preserved. While the 15% reduction in calories may not total one pound in a week, it could add up to one pound in 2 weeks or one pound in 10 days and most of the weight loss will be fat, not muscle. Ideally, Jane should make a reduction of 15% or 270 calories.

Q: If I burn 3500 calories a week through exercise will I lose a pound of fat in a week?

A: Yes, expending 3500 calories will lead to a pound of fat loss. However, you can still burn some fat, without any change in your caloric intake, by burning less than 3500 calories a week. If you walk for an hour, you may burn off 200 to 250 calories. Although it would take a bit more than 2 weeks to burn the pound of fat, it may be better for you in the long run because a more involved exercise program may be hard to sustain and slow weight loss is always the way to go, as most of the weight loss on a slower weight loss program will be derived from body fat stores, not muscle stores.

Q: How about exercise and dieting? Isn't that the best way to go?

A: Exercise and dieting at the same time may lead to faster progress, but many find it too overwhelming-committing to daily exercise and recording food consumption-at the same time. For many, the best results may come from dieting alone or from exercising with no change in eating habits. Exercise will also help in preserving lean body mass (muscle), which revs the metabolism.

When embarking upon a diet and exercise program, 3500 calories can be burned off/deleted from the diet so a pound of fat can be burned. To create a deficit of 3500 calories in 10 days, you should create a 350 calorie deficit each day (3500/10). Ideally, this can be done by splitting the 350 calories in two. One hundred and seventy-five calories will have to be expended through exercise each day and you will have to eat 175 less calories a day.

It may be surprising to you that such small alterations in your life can lead to weight loss. This is why it is important to keep a food record of all the foods you eat every day. It is very hard to eyeball 175 calories and it is very easy to have an extra 175 calories, or even an additional 500 calories sneak into your diet unless you really know exactly what you are eating.

Many reject the idea of becoming a food accountant, recording every item of food eaten each day. Instead, they opt to haphazardly cut calories or to make a large cut hoping for their bodies to respond. Losing fat weight and keeping it off requires willpower, knowledge, and action. Many have the will, this book will give you the knowledge, but only you have the final say. Unless you commit yourself, are dedicated, and keep records all your willpower and dedication will be wasted.

Chapter Nine

Alternative Diet Strategies
Eating At Night: Rights and Wrongs

Bodybuilders are some of the leanest people on earth. In an attempt to shed every ounce of excessive fat, bodybuilders often stop eating late at night. Specifically, many will reduce their carbohydrate intake as the day progresses in hope that more fat will be lost.

I've heard it over and over again, "If you want to get lean, cut your carbs out completely after 4 PM." Others suggest 6 PM and I have heard as early as 3 PM on several occasions. Maybe someone you know has suggested the same. While reducing carbohydrates late in the day may be helpful in losing fat, other important factors need to be taken into consideration as well. My experience has shown that eating carbohydrates at night, under certain circumstances, cause you to store calories as fat. Carbohydrates seem to pose a special problem for those seeking low body fat levels. After all, carbohydrates are the chief fuel of source for working muscles. You need them while working out with weights to increase muscle mass and adding muscle is the real way to increase your metabolism. Eating too few, especially over a period of three to four days, could lead to muscular fatigue. On the other hand, carbohydrates, especially when eaten in excess, have the potential to stimulate fat storage.

Carbs and Fat Control

The primary rule in controlling body fat is to prevent the body from storing fat in the first place (see Chapter 4: **Fat Inhibition**). Avoiding an excessive caloric intake, yet eating within your daily caloric needs is a must if you hope to attain a low level of body fat. To lose fat, energy from calories must be reduced or calories must be expended through exercise. When the body perceives a caloric deficit, it will be forced to use a greater degree of body fat as fuel. Be careful, too large a deficit will cause the body to fight back by hoarding fat.

While reducing calories is an important step in controlling body fat, other factors also play a role in initiating fat storage. Low fiber diets can lead to overeating, and a high sugar and high fat diet can increase the fat storing machinery without you eating a calorie excess.

With this in mind, I have noticed that an excess of refined sugars such as fruit juice and honey, or carbohydrates that lack fiber like white rice, mashed potatoes and cold breakfast cereals tend to break down in the body too fast. When carbohydrates are rapidly digested, sugar, in the form of glucose, derived from the carbohydrate foods, floods the blood stream and elicits a larger output of the hormone insulin. This hormone's main function is to regulate glucose (blood sugar) levels. It does so by transporting glucose to all the body's cells where it can be called upon to provide fuel. One of the major storage units for sugar is muscle glycogen. Although glycogen can be readily accessed to provide energy, the body's cells can become saturated, and any excess sugar will be stored as fat. Essentially, the amount of glycogen already stored in muscle constitutes the main factor as to the fate of those carbohydrates. Thus, controlling the amount of carbohydrates ingested while eating a low fat, high fiber, low sugar, and calorically balanced diet (calorically balanced accounts for your BM plus activity) is a key in achieving low fat and preventing fat storage.

I believe that one way to control glucose levels and the associated probability of fat storage is to avoid a high carbohydrate intake later in the evening. While total calories are probably most important in the fate of body fat levels, lowering glucose levels by avoiding late night meals may also play a strong role. Foods consumed later in the night have a greater tendency to be stored as fat for three reasons:

1) You are less active at night and caloric expenditure is lower.

2) Your carbohydrate stores (as glycogen) may be sufficiently full from eating through the day, so more carbs = more fat.

3) Carbohydrates cause more insulin release at night versus in the morning. Three hundred calories worth of potatoes at 7 PM will cause more insulin release than the same 300 calories worth of potatoes eaten at 7 AM.

Cutting Carbs For Fat Loss

By now, you probably understand my strong bias in choosing weight training as a long term fat burner over aerobic exercise. Weight training is really the way to go for revving the metabolism. The information below pertains to the person who chooses weight training as his mode of exercise for calorie expenditure. If you are still unsure why I put weight training on a pedestal, go back and read Chapter 5.

If you are exercising with weights earlier in the day, then you should continue with a larger post training meal, but your final meal should be lower in carbohydrates. The latter will allow for optimal (natural) growth hormone release and lowering carbohydrates will enhance the body's natural use of fat as fuel. When carbohydrate reserves as glycogen are not full and blood sugar levels are on the lower side, fat is more readily broken down from fat reserves to be used as fuel.

The net insulin released is correlated to many factors. The main insulin releaser is total carbohydrate intake and a close second is sugar filled, refined or simple carbohydrates.

Obese individuals have insulin receptors on fat cells that are very active. Correspondingly, the receptors on muscle tissue are less active.

In the person who is lean and has a high BM due to plenty of muscle mass, the receptors for insulin on fat cells are much less active *because* the receptors for insulin on muscle cells are extremely active.

How does this apply to you? Allow me to elucidate. If your goal is to control body fat first, or if you have a difficult time losing fat, then it may be a good idea to curtail your carbohydrate intake at night and to make sure you are not overeating carbohydrates, in total, each day. Remember, once glycogen stores are full, extra carbs can store as fat and insulin levels are higher at night. (high insulin can store fat)

If you are lean, then you probably can eat more of your total carbohydrates for the day later in the day because muscles that are sensitive to insulin will use the sugar (as long as your calories are not excessive) as fuel.

As body fat levels drop, you can then eat some more of your carbohydrates later in the day without storing them because with a decrease in body fat, you will also experience a slightly lower output in insulin in response to carbohydrate foods.

If you have not cut calories and are trying to burn fat by adding lean body mass and are training with weights after work in the evening, then it is important to eat more of your carbohydrates at night after training.

Before going on, it is important for you to grasp an important concept. Muscles have active receptors to insulin. When muscles have been worked, the receptors for insulin work overtime. When carbohydrates are consumed when these receptors are "turned on high" the body does not have to release as much insulin. Sugar deprived muscles (as a result of a hard training session) will "draw" the attention of insulin towards them and store sugars, from carbohydrates, as muscle glycogen. *If carbs are headed towards muscle then they are not headed towards fat.*

If you are following a training program to build muscle to "build" your metabolism, and you are not altering your caloric intake, it is vitally important to eat more of your daily allotment of carbohydrates after training as they will restore muscle glycogen since glycogen stores are lowered with training and receptors for insulin is higher after training. The carbohydrates at this time have a very little chance to be stored as fat.

Don't make the mistake of cutting carbohydrates in the evening if you trained with weights. This will lead to lower muscle recovery, so the adaptation process of adding muscle mass, the process that is so effective in kicking up the metabolism will be hindered. If you are training with weights in the morning hours, then the meal following training should be higher in carbohydrates, but your last meal should be lower in carbohydrates.

Growth Hormone: **A Sparkplug For Fat Loss**

Another reason to avoid late night carbohydrate intake or to lower carbohydrate intake in the later hours is to harness the body's output of growth hormone. Growth hormone is released at night within the first 60 minutes of deep sleep. Growth hormone is beneficial to a person who wishes to shed fat and hold muscle as growth hormone causes the body to burn more fat instead of burning lean body mass. Growth hormone initiates a moderate shifting in fuel sources so the body burns more fatty acids at rest at the expense of burning less glycogen and especially body protein. The net result of taking advantage of your body's output of growth hormone is additional fat loss without losing muscle mass. Losing muscle mass can defeat the purpose of dieting as a lower amount of muscle is directly tied to a lower metabolism. A person who diets and has a slow metabolism will see few results and quit any diet due to a lack of results.

Carbohydrates consumed before going off to bed can

blunt the body's natural release of this hormone because high blood sugar levels inhibit growth hormone release while low levels obtained from avoiding or lowering carbohydrate intake at this time can increase and facilitate the release of this fat burning hormone.

For those who eat a higher carb intake after training in the evening, don't you worry. Carbohydrates, introduced to muscles that have just finished exercising with weights, will be quickly removed from the blood and enter the muscle as glycogen to replenish glycogen stores to support muscle recovery. This leaves blood sugar levels low so growth hormone can be released.

We can apply this strategy to our example of the woman who, with the use of weight training, increased her lean body mass from 127 pounds to 137 pounds.

She was eating 137 grams of protein a day split into 6 meals yielding 23 grams of protein at each meal along with 187 grams of carbohydrates a day which is equivalent to 31 grams of carbohydrates at each meal.

She can take advantage of the fact that carbohydrates can be more readily stored at night by adjusting her carbohydrates as so:

Original carbohydrate intake: New carb intake:

Meal 1 31 grams	Meal 1 37 grams	
Meal 2 31 grams	Meal 2 37 grams	
Meal 3 31 grams	Meal 3 37 grams	
Meal 4 31 grams	Meal 4 21 grams	allows for a
Meal 5 31 grams	Meal 5 21 grams	lower BS level
Meal 6 31 grams	Meal 6 21 grams	at night

In the example above, I just took 10 grams of carbs from the final three meals and added them to the first three meals. Here, she will be active during the day and has a good chance of burning the carbohydrates off as fuel as the day progresses. Plus, her allotment for carbohydrates (187) is not exceeded.

If she is training, I suggest that 25% of the day's allotment of carbohydrates be consumed in the morning at breakfast where blood sugar levels are low due to an overnight "fast" of sorts and another 25% of the total carbohydrate intake be relegated to the meal following a weight training session.

Here's how it looks:

25% of 187 is approximately 47 grams of
    carbohydrates
47 gm (at breakfast) + 47 gm (after training) =
    94 grams
187 (total carb allotment) - 94 gm (at two meals) =
    93 grams
93 gm (remaining) divided by 4 meals (remaining) =
    23 grams/meal

Original Carb Intake: Carb Intake with Training:

Meal 1	31 gram	Meal 1	47 grams
Meal 2	31 grams	Meal 2	23 grams*
Meal 3	31 grams	Meal 3	23 grams*
Meal 4	31 grams	Meal 4	23 grams*
Meal 5	31 grams	Meal 5	23 grams*
Meal 6	31 grams		-Train With Weights-
		Meal 6	47 grams

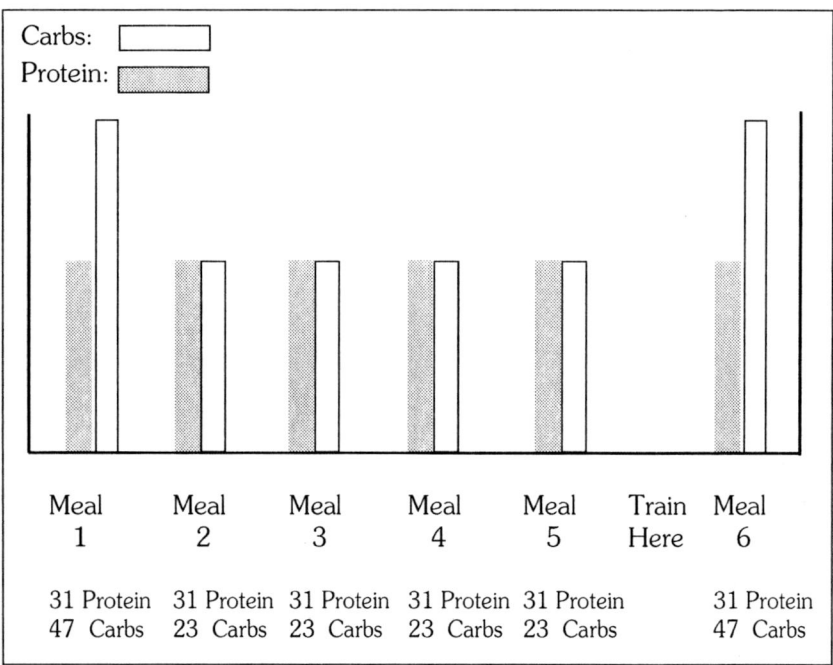

Carbs:
Protein:

Meal 1	Meal 2	Meal 3	Meal 4	Meal 5	Train Here	Meal 6
31 Protein	31 Protein	31 Protein	31 Protein	31 Protein		31 Protein
47 Carbs	23 Carbs	23 Carbs	23 Carbs	23 Carbs		47 Carbs

* At these times, blood sugar levels are lower, probably closer to the 70 (see page 26). Any time blood sugar levels fall, the body will release opposing hormones to increase blood sugar levels. These hormones, glucagon and epinephrine, cause the body to mobilize fat stores as well.

This is yet another way to promote fat loss or to initiate fat breakdown without cutting calories, without any major change in diet, and without the use of drastic measures which can slow the metabolism and make weight loss extremely difficult and discouraging.

Comparative Between Original Carb Intake and Carb Intake With Training and a Large Breakfast

MEAL 1   becomes...   MEAL 1
1 1/2 oz. oatmeal   2 1/2 oz. oatmeal

MEAL 2   becomes...   MEAL 2
1 1/2 oz. pasta w/   1 oz. pasta w/
   small salad   small salad

MEAL 3   becomes...   MEAL 3
cup rice   2/3 cup rice

MEAL 4   becomes...   MEAL 4
pita   2/3 pita

MEAL 5   becomes...   MEAL 5
2 cups yogurt   1 cup yogurt w/
                                    1/4 cup non fat
                                    cottage cheese

MEAL 6   becomes...   MEAL 6
5 oz. potato w/   7.5 oz. potato w/
   salad   salad

Chapter Ten

Low Carb Diets For The Obese

Over the past ten years, a low fat diet that emphasizes plenty of energy rich complex carbohydrates has been the diet regiment that Americans have adopted in a quest for a fat free body. Combined with exercise, a high carbohydrate diet, one that includes foods like potatoes, yams, whole grain rice, whole grain breads, beans, and fruit has been used by millions to reduce fat stores. However, during the same time, the nation as a whole has become fatter than ever.

Many who successfully subscribe to the high carbohydrate diet believe a low carb approach to fat loss is dietary suicide. For those of you who have failed to attain a low level of body fat using a high carbohydrate diet, and for those who have exercised religiously, hour upon hour, week after week, and failed to attain a "six-pack-rack" of abdominals, hard glutes, and a low level of body fat, the low carb approach may be suited for you. For the obese, who have over 50 pounds of fat to lose, this may also be an alternative that will work.

The low carb diet is considered by many to be an extreme approach to fat loss. However, it is an easy diet to follow and may be much easier for you if you can't stand the thought of becoming a food accountant-weighing foods, measuring, reading every label and taking records. While I actually enjoy doing this, many are overwhelmed and find counting carbohydrates, and carbohydrates alone, an easy way to achieve their weight loss goals.

A high carbohydrate, moderate protein, low fat diet will work for some, but for others, it is a futile effort, a false promise.

For those who are still too soft, for the obese, and for those who feel the high carb diet failed, here is an alternative that can work for you.

We already know carbs are required by the body but an excess can be stored as fat. I also told you about the rats injected with insulin that ate until their stomachs exploded. And insulin can inhibit hormone sensitive lipase, the enzyme that allows fat cells to release fat while increasing the amount of lipoprotein lipase in the body, the cousin to hormone sensitive lipase. Lipoprotein lipase causes fat cells to store fat. These factors are especially true in obese individuals and may be true in people who have been fat, or borderline obese, for years.

It seems that a good diet that matches BM and activity levels may not work for the obese and others. Reducing calories may not work. The body simply adjusts to the cut with speed, accuracy, and precision. Exercise can be too difficult as it can be hard to move around such a large mass.

The only way to initiate fat burning may be to resort to the extreme. In this case, the extreme is a very low carbohydrate diet. Cutting carbohydrates completely from the diet, no bread, no sugar, no potatoes, pasta, rice, cereal, etc. will drastically lower blood sugar levels. When blood sugar levels stay low for an extended period of time, more than five days, a cascade of hormonal reactions occur that favor fat burning.

In between meals, when carbohydrate intake is curtailed or when carbohydrates intake is restricted, the body releases opposing hormones that raise sugar levels in the blood. Glucagon from the pancreas and epinephrine from the adrenals, raise blood sugar levels by initiating the liver to breakdown stored muscle glycogen. Glycogen, the storage form of glucose, is subsequently sent back into glucose, to increase sugar levels in the blood. (see drawing)

1)

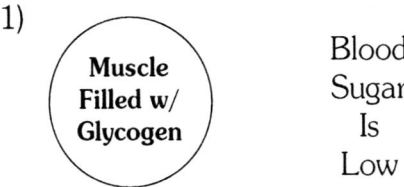

Blood
Sugar
Is
Low

2) Glucagon, epinephrine, hormone sensitive lipase
released causing:

3)

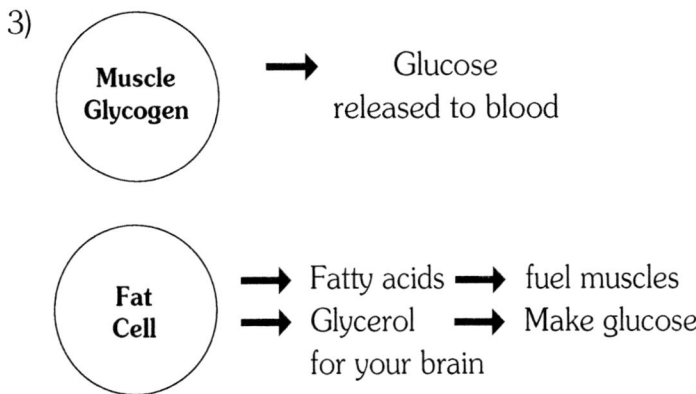

Epinephrine, and to a lesser degree, glucagon, stimulate lipolysis, fat breakdown from fat cells. Fat cells are made of fatty acids and glycerol. The fatty acids liberated as a result of low blood sugar levels, can be used by muscles, and glycerol can be used by the liver to make glucose to feed the brain and heart. So far, so good. The net effect of low blood sugar is an increase in fat mobilization!

Second Stringers

When the body is subjected to long periods of low blood sugar, the body releases growth hormone and cortisol. Growth hormone causes fat cells to break down, so more fatty acids and glycerol can be released to fuel muscles and the brain. Cortisol is required for growth hormone to work its fat liberating magic on fat cells.

Muscle Wastage

The drawback to a low carb diet is the potential for muscle loss, as the hormone insulin is needed to drive amino acids from protein foods into the muscles and cortisol causes the muscles to break down so amino acids, that comprise muscle tissue, can be used to be converted into sugar.

This muscle loss can be significantly slowed in two ways. GH is released with a prolonged low blood sugar level and causes more fat to be broken down for fuel. It also prevents muscles to be broken down. In fact GH increases the uptake of amino acids by muscles. This amino acid uptake could combat the negative muscle wasting effects of cortisol.

Increasing the intake of dietary protein when carbohydrates are reduced will spare the body from tearing apart muscle tissue to be used as glucose. This increase in protein consumption will allow the body to convert the protein in the blood (from foods) into new glucose instead of tearing down muscle to obtain similar amino acids. Increasing your protein intake is essential while lowering carbohydrate intake and total calorie intake. Additional protein, up to 1.5 grams per pound of lean body mass was necessary to maintain body protein in studies with obese patients. Eskimos, who eat a strictly meat diet, one that yields essentially zero carbohydrates, consume at least double the amount of protein compared to the RDA.

Ketones...A Litmus Test For Fat Metabolism

Lowering your carbohydrate intake along with a low fat and higher protein diet is, like any diet, a modified form of fasting. When fuel intakes decrease, the body taps other sources of fuel. After the body's stores of carbohydrate are essentially used up in two to five days, the body begins to tap significantly more body fat, and to a lesser extent, more body protein.

As fat is broken down, the fatty acids are sent to the liver to make a special molecule called acetyl coenzyme A, an intermediary in fat metabolism. When fat metabolism is peaking, so much fat is being broken down, and so much acetyl CoA forms, that the body responds by bundling together the acetate molecules of acetyl CoA and produces ketones. Excess ketones leak out of the liver and flow out of the blood and are excreted in the urine. Ketones that are not excreted enter the blood and are used by the brain for fuel, which spares glucose (the brain can only use glucose and ketones for fuel, not fat!). Muscles also use ketones as fuel. I find ketones to be a powerful alternative fuel source which allow fat derived calories to power the brain. When ketones are made, the body does not have to make as much glucose from body protein to feed the brain. Therefore, ketones are protein sparing. Ketones can have protein (muscle) sparing effects on obese patients who follow starvation type diets.

Protein and Carb Requirements
On A Low Carb Diet

When carbohydrates are reduced, and glycogen stores are very low, and fat metabolism is in high gear, protein is broken down to make new glucose which is used to feed the brain. If a person eats no carbohydrates at all, the body can use up to 200 grams of protein daily just to feed the brain. My recommendation is to first limit insulin release by cutting carbs to 50 or 100 grams a day. This small amount of carbohydrates will be used to fuel the brain (50) and if you are working out, give yourself another 50 grams, for a total of 100. Lowering blood sugar levels by limiting carbohydrates will stimulate the fat mobilizing effects of glucagon, epinephrine, GH, cortisol, and ketones.

Protein must remain high as dietary protein, supplied in higher amounts, can offset some of the muscle wasting effects associated with any reducing program. On a low carb diet, I suggest 1.5 grams of protein for each pound of your goal weight. If you weigh 178 and wish to reduce to 158, your protein intake should be approximately 237 grams a day. If you work out, or on days you train with weights, your protein intake can rise to 2 grams per pound of goal weight. If you are a bodybuilder and carry lots of muscle, you will need more protein, as high as 2.5 to 3 grams for each pound of goal weight.

Ketostix, purchased in any pharmacy, can quickly inform you if you are in ketosis. It is possible to be burning body fat without the test showing you have ketones in the urine as it is excess ketones that spill from the liver and enter the urine that gives an indication of ketosis. If your test reads negative ketones, then continue with the low carb diet plan and shoot for a weight loss of one to two pounds a week.

If you do reach ketosis, I suggest you stay in it for no more than three days in a row. Then, lower your protein intake to .5 grams of protein per goal weight if you are inactive and 1 gram of protein per pound of goal weight if you are training with weights or if you are bodybuilding. At the same time increase your carbohydrate intake to 2 grams of carbs per goal weight if you are inactive, and 3 grams of carbs per goal weight if you are active or bodybuilding. Keep the carbohydrates higher for 1 day then go back to the lower carbohydrate intake. Upping your carb intake will do two things. It will put an abrupt end to ketone (over) production so ketones will no longer be found in the urine. Second, increasing carbohydrates can offset a metabolic slowdown. When calories and carbs are lowered, the body can react by slowing its output of the hormone called thyroid. Thyroid is intricately involved in fat metabolism and calorie burning. Low levels are detrimental to calorie burning. Adding in a high amount of carbs, when ketone production is in high gear, can trick the body, causing it to continue to release thyroid instead of slowing its output. The effect is normal thyroid levels to keep calorie burning high while calories are reduced which causes fat breakdown.

Ketones are naturally safe. It is excessive ketones, ketosis for too long, that could lead to acidosis in the blood, a dangerous problem which is mainly associated with diabetics. Diabetic acidosis, I feel, has given ketone bodies a bad and unfair reputation.

No Fat Needed

Some authors, dieticians, and books claim those who restrict carbohydrates can indulge in high fat foods, bacon, ham, sausage, whole eggs, and steaks, and not gain fat, because insulin is the "sparkplug" that promotes dietary fat to be stored. This is false. While high insulin is the sparkplug that can store fat, eating too much fat provides the building blocks, fatty acids and glycerol, that can be used to make body fat. Eating fat can provide fatty acids that can be used by muscles as fuel and glycerol can be converted to glucose to feed the brain. My simple question is this. Why add extra dietary fat to the diet if the body can readily break apart body fat to obtain the same substrates (fat and glycerol) *especially if fat reduction is the main goal?*

Sample 5 Meal Plan for a Non Training Person:
Weight: 178 lbs.
Goal: 158 lbs.*

* Goal weight is approximate to Lean Body Mass.

237 grams of protein and 50 grams of carbohydrates....
All meals yield approximately 47 grams of protein
  (47 x 5 = 235)

Protein		Carbohydrates (50)
Meal 1	15 egg whites	1 slice bread
Meal 2	10 oz. chicken breast	0
Meal 3	10 oz. steak	3 rice cakes
Meal 4	9 oz. turkey breast	salad
Meal 5	12 oz. fish	salad

HIGH CARBOHYDRATE DAY

Carbohydrate Intake Should Be:
158 x 2 = 316 carbohydrates which is approximately
        63 grams each meal

Protein Intake Should Be:
158 x (.5) = approximately 80 which is
        16 grams per meal

Protein		Carbohydrates	
Meal 1	5 egg whites	3 slices whole grain bread	
Meal 2	3 oz. chicken (PCW)	3 oz. pasta (PCW)	
Meal 3	3 oz. steak (PCW)	2 cups rice, cooked	
Meal 4	4 oz. fish (PCW)	10 oz. potato (PCW)	
Meal 5	3 oz. chicken (PCW)	10 oz. yam (PCW)	

PCW= "pre cooked weight"

Chapter Eleven

Thermogenesis: Heat Production For Fat Loss

Thermogenesis is a fancy word for heat. The normal body temperature is 98.6 F. Every time fuel is introduced into the body from foods, the body temperature rises to a small degree.

Thermogenesis is formerly known as the SDA effect or the specific dynamic action effect. SDA/thermogenesis concludes that carbohydrates, protein, and fat cause unique increases in heat production.

If you can get your body to produce more heat, then more of the energy from the calories you eat will simply be "burned off" as heat. This leaves less net calories (from the food) available to be used as fuel. The fate of these calories (as fuel) can be burned to provide energy to the body or they can be stored as glycogen or fat.

Some nutrients exert a higher thermic (heat producing effect) than others. Protein exerts the strongest thermic effect, carbohydrate exert a milder effect, but dietary fat exerts a very minute dietary induced thermic effect. One reason 100 calories of dietary fat has an easier tendency to be stored as fat when compared to 100 calories of carbs is due to thermogenesis. Fat is only 3% thermic. When you eat 100 calories of fat, 3 of the 100 calories will be burned off immediately as heat. When you eat 100 calories of carbohydrates, 12 to 15 of the 100 calories of carbohydrates will immediately "wasted" as heat.

Dietary induced thermogenesis occurs to a greater degree in lean individuals. The more fat you carry the less thermogenesis occurs in your body. Fat acts as an insulator. It traps heat. When it is really cold outside and you want to remain warm, you throw on a big-oversized-warm jacket. That jacket will trap heat inside so heat cannot escape. Body fat acts as nature's jacket. It traps heat so your body heat is less likely to escape.

Those who have less fat experience greater thermic effects from foods. With less insulation, more heat can escape. When more heat escapes, the body compensates by generating more heat inside the body to make up for the lost heat.

Diets that reduce thermogenesis include:
1) Low protein diets
2) Low carbohydrate diets
3) High fat diets
4) Low salt diets

When calories are too low as common with dieting, the body produces less heat. When the body temperature falls, less total calories are burned at rest. No wonder low calorie diets fail.

One reason people who eat a low fat diet find dieting to be more successful, is due to the low thermic effect of fat. When calories are reduced by a small margin and fat is reduced while carbohydrates and protein are kept at adequate levels, the body can tap fat as fuel without decreasing its thermic effect.

Interestingly, a low carbohydrate diet can fail because low carb diets are correlated with a lower thermic effect. However, a low carb diet with increased amounts of protein in the diet may offset the lowered thermic effect associated with a low carb diet as protein exerts a strong thermic effect.

Diets that increase thermogenesis include

1) Diets that are adequate in calories (i.e. match your BM and activity levels).
2) Diets that are above calorie requirements.
3) Diets that include frequent feedings.

Excess calories increase thermogenesis, especially when the excess calories come from carbohydrates. Although eating excess carbohydrates will increase heat production, body fat can readily be stored with a caloric excess. If more calories are introduced to the body than burned off as metabolic heat, thermic heat, or exercise, fat is deposited. However, an increase in calories that causes an increase in thermogenesis may also explain why a person who continues to overeat will reach a point and not get significantly fatter. The more he overeats, the more heat is produced. Think of it this way. When calories are reduced, fat is given up as fuel. When calories are radically reduced, you would expect body fat to be shed at record speed. But the opposite occurs. Severe dieting causes a metabolic slowdown through a loss of muscle mass and a marked decrease in both body temperature and heat production induced by foods. If you cut 1200 calories from your diet you would expect a 3 pound fat loss in 3 days (3 x 1200 = 3600 calories and a pound of fat = 3500 calories). In reality, three pounds is not lost due to a slower metabolism, lowered body temperature and lowered dietary induced thermogenesis. At the other end of the spectrum, the person who overeats, especially if those foods are made of complex carbohydrates and lean proteins that are not high in fat, will experience greater thermogenesis. Both his body temperature and the heat produced from foods will be at its peak. This helps to explain why a person who overeats 1200 calories a day for three days does not gain a pound of fat. He may gain fat, but it may be less than expected. Perhaps 1/2 or 3/4 of a pound is gained, but not the full pound.

How does this apply to you? If you are going to overeat, choose complex carbs (not sugary carbs) and lean proteins.

Another reason to split your daily calories in 4, 5 or even six meals is to harness your body's natural thermic ability. Every time you eat, thermogenesis is turned on, so it makes sense to turn it on as many times as you can while eating within your daily caloric requirements.

Americans are obsessed with eating low fat. That's great. But, many break lots of dietary rules that can promote fat storage while still eating low fat. The mistakes they make include

1) eating only 2 to 3 times a day
2) not eating sufficient fiber
3) eating too many fast acting (simple) carbs
4) eating too many of their total calories at night
5) not eating enough at breakfast

And now, we are drastically lowering our intake of salt. Last year, ABC NEWS ran a segment that challenged the government's recommendation that

Americans eat less salt as high salt can cause an increase in blood pressure. The piece raised very strong doubts that salt is the culprit in high blood pressure and even stronger doubts were expressed as to whether salt is correlated with heart disease. Now, we have a country that diets on very low calories in an attempt to shed fat and avoids salt like the plaque because everyone says it's bad.

While there is more information out there among the masses as to the smart way to lose fat and there are millions following this good advice, there are more people than ever following very low calorie diets. Low calorie diets lower metabolism and heat production and now I inform you that diets low in salt can also decrease heat production!

Salt contains iodine, the mineral that helps regulate the thyroid hormone. Thyroid hormones play an important role in calorie burning. When iodine levels are too low, as can be found with a zero salt diet, thyroid levels can fall, making weight loss and thermogenesis lower.

Thermogenesis also works with exercise. *Exercise induced thermogenesis* occurs in muscle. When you exercise to burn calories, some of the calories burned come from doing the work. But, some calories are burned when the body temperature rises causing you to sweat. My guess is that exercising with too much clothing could trap heat in the body reducing exercise induced thermogenesis.

Chapter Twelve

Exercise: A Closer Look

Thus far, my main emphasis has been on diet and body fat. While I have touched upon exercise as a means to burn some calories in weight loss, I haven't been so specific.

Exercise burns calories. If you can burn more calories, without eating additional food, the body will give up stored body fat as a fuel source.

I already showed you how the body adapts to aerobic exercise, now I want to show you a few more differences between aerobic exercise and weight training (anaerobic exercise).

When a person begins a stringent weight loss program with diet alone, a combination of body fat and lean muscle mass is burned. With severe caloric reductions *an equal amount of muscle and fat could be lost!* The result could be a person who lost 50 pounds, lost 25 pounds of muscle and the same amount of fat. While he now weighs less his body fat percentage has not changed.

A person who adds cardio work to a severe caloric

reduction may lose weight faster and may lose more. The person who combines aerobic exercise with a severe diet could lose 55 pounds, but 22 of those pounds is still muscle. With a severe diet or with a severe diet combined with aerobic exercise, muscle is wasted away as the body breaks down muscles to obtain amino acids which it can change into glucose (fuel). Aerobic exercise will burn more calories, but it will fail to prevent the body from tearing down muscle.

When weight resistance exercises are added to a severe diet, the body may shed the same 50 pounds, but approximately 75% will come from fat stores. Adding resistance to muscles will cause some muscle preservation so less muscle is torn apart.

Therefore, as three different people lose approximately 50 pounds each, the person who trained with weights will be far better off as he has saved some of his muscle and we know that muscle has the single greatest effect on the metabolism.

Person A: Severe Diet
Person B: Severe Diet and Aerobic Exercise
Person C: Severe Diet and Weight Training

Start Weight	End Weight	Fat Loss	Muscle Loss	Effect on Metabolism
A) 250	200	25 lbs.	25 lbs.	slowest
B) 250	200	28	22	slower
C) 250	200	35	15	slow

As you can see, weight training acts as the stimulus to cause the body to hold muscle tissue. Thus, it is better than aerobic exercise as a tool in altering body fat levels because the more muscle you have, the faster or higher the metabolism.

In fact, a higher metabolism, which is created by adding muscle mass through weight training, is more important than exercise itself in keeping your body fat levels under control and in check.

Refer back to page 39 when I provided an easy formula for outlining the amount of calories your body needed in a day. The BM (basal metabolism) the amount of calories you need every day even at rest and doing absolutely nothing at all will use more calories than heavy exercise. A person with 180 pounds of muscle mass will require 1800 calories a day sitting at home and watching television all day. It would take him three hours of very intensive exercise to burn off that amount, or he could go for a long leisurely walk about-oh-12 miles!!

The way to lose fat and to keep the metabolism from slowing is through a diet that provides a very small deficit in calories to initiate fat breakdown. Then, you must add weight training to build the metabolism. Everyone will lose more fat than muscle on such a program. If you want to burn additional calories, an aerobic program can be used, but don't rely on aerobics exclusively. As far as exercise, place the most emphasis on building the muscle with weight training. Use some aerobic exercise to burn some additional calories. I think three 20 to 30 minute aerobic sessions each week is suffice to help cause weight loss in addition to your weight training workouts. Remember, more aerobics *is not better*, just as less calories *will not* cause the body to speed up weight loss. The body runs on checks and balances and it will adapt to sharp caloric restrictions by slowing its metabolism and large amount of aerobic exercise by becoming efficient by burning less calories when performing the (aerobic) exercise.

High Intensity Aerobics Is Better

Aerobic exercise makes use of large muscle groups in a rhythmic sustained fashion. Aerobic exercise elevates and maintains a consistent heart rate for 20 minutes or more. One way the body adapts to this type of exercise is by strengthening and improving the function and efficiency of the heart and lungs. More popular activities include brisk walking, jogging, cycling, swimming, or stair climbing (machines). The fuel for sustained exercise is fat. Therefore this type of exercise can burn calories in the form of stored body fat and it can improve overall health.

One special adaptation at the cellular level is an increase in the size of the mitochondria. The mitochondria is the muscles cell's "powerhouse." When calories are reduced or when a person exercises and fat is broken down, the fatty acids derived from stored body fat are burned as fuel in the "powerhouse." Aerobic exercise can increase the size of the powerhouse, so fat can be more readily and efficiently burned. The mitochondria could be considered the end of the line in the fat burning process. Enlarging your "powerhouses" can make fat loss easier.

Many ask me what type of aerobic exercise is better? High intensity or lower intensity?

The answer is high intensity. Aerobic intensity is measured by your heart rate. The harder the exercise, the more our heart works and the more your heart works, the more calories are burned.

Most recommend cardiovascular enthusiasts exercise in their "target heart rate." To find target heart rate, minus your age from 220 and multiply by .60 to .75. I am 30 years old, so the numbers look like so.

$$220 - 30 = 190 \text{ beats}$$

190 x .60 = 114 beats in one minute
190 x .75 = 142 beats in one minute

Here is a target heart rate table. Match your age to the heart rates below.

Heart Rate at age . . .	60%	70%	75%
20	120	140	150
25	117	137	146
30	114	133	142
35	111	130	139
40	108	126	135
45	105	123	131
50	102	119	128
55	99	116	124
60	96	112	120
65	93	109	116
70	90	105	113

(heart rates in beats per minute)

For those who are trying to get in shape for the first time and for those who have more than 30 pounds of fat to lose, I recommend a lower level of intensity. If you are extremely out of shape, you can exercise at an even lower level, a 50% heart rate until the exercise becomes easier for you. Then you can up the intensity. When performing the aerobic work, shoot for 60% of your target heart rate.

Aerobic exercise earned its respect in the weight loss community because it definitely burns calories, it can improve fat burning efficiency by increasing the size of the mitochondria, and most important, the fuel source for the exercise is fat! Thus, aerobics has been the preferred form of exercise for weight control.

To harness these benefits, one should engage in three times a week exercise sessions. I don't think more is better. As far as exercise, I suggest that you first concentrate on building the metabolism with weight training, then use aerobic exercise as a way to burn additional calories and to improve the body's ability to burn fat (by increasing the size of the mitochondria).

However, if you are more than 30 pounds over your goal weight and you tire easy and experience shortness of breath, I suggest you emphasize the right diet first. Choose a diet that creates a small caloric deficit, then build your strength slowly with some aerobic exercise. After weight loss has begun, and you feel more energetic and stronger throughout the day, you can begin a weight training program.

Best Time To Exercise

Is there a best time to exercise? Yes. A body burns a greater amount of fat when it is exercised in the morning compared to the afternoon. Aerobic exercise is more effective at breaking down stored fat as fuel when performed in the morning without eating.

Aerobics taps fat as fuel. When a person eats a carbohydrate snack, before performing aerobic exercise, the carbohydrates will release insulin which opposes fat breakdown. Once a person has been performing an exercise for more than 3 to 5 minutes, the body will normally shift fuel sources so more fat is used. During the first 3 to 5 minutes more glucose is used from stored glycogen and from the glucose found in the blood. Although the body will shift fuel sources after 3 to 5 minutes, you have sent a signal, via insulin, to disallow or at least fight, the signal being sent with continuous aerobic exercise. Fat may still be used, but I doubt to the degree that an empty stomach training session would generate.

If you want to burn fat with aerobic exercise, perform your exercise on an empty stomach first thing in the morning. When blood sugar levels are lower in the morning and remain low by avoiding food, the body will quickly look for fat to fuel the workouts.

Chapter Thirteen

Genetics and Bodyfat

Unquestionably, genetics play a role in the amount of fat cells a person has and his ability to both deposit calories as fat or liberate fat from storage.

Your genes play a big role in determining your success in body fat control. If one parent is overweight, a child has a 40% chance of becoming obese. If both parents are obese, the odds increase to 60%. The total number of fat cells found on the body is influenced by three factors:

1) the amount of fat cells the biological parents have
2) the amount of weight the mother gains while pregnant, especially during the last trimester
3) the amount of fat gained during the teenage years

As you can see, you will have to work extra hard and extra smart with your nutrition and exercise if one or both of your parents were overweight. If you gained a lot of fat as a teenager, weight loss may be more difficult. An overweight teenager will have a 60% to 70% chance of staying obese throughout life. All three contribute to more fat cells.

If a person has *more* fat cells than another, he can appear much fatter even if the fat cells that he has are not enlarged. If a person has *very few* fat cells, but those fat cells are relatively full, he will be *leaner* than the former.

When a person has a large number of fat cells, these cells are more sensitive to insulin, they have high amounts of the fat storing enzyme lipoprotein lipase, there is an increased ability to manufacture fatty acids from glucose, and overall, the fat cell is really good at storing fat. While diet and exercise will absolutely reduce fat stores and make a genetically fat person leaner, the shrunken fat cells retain ALL of its fat storing capabilities, so anytime there is a lapse in either exercise of diet, the body will rapidly store fat at a rate that is efficient and dramatically faster than a person who is the offspring of two lean parents. When a person becomes obese, he changes his body chemistry so fat storage is always favored. This helps to explain why millions can lose 20, 40, 80 or over 200 pounds and gain it all back again.

If, both parents are lean, and the mother didn't gain an excessive amount of weight in the third trimester of pregnancy, then a child will more than likely be born with a normal or lower amount of total fat cells. A lean individual (via genetics) who eats low fat, high-fiber foods devoid of sugar will have a very different genetic fat storing chemistry. Insulin levels are lower, lipoprotein lipase is less active at the expense of the fat liberating enzyme hormone sensitive lipase, thermogenesis imparts its full effect and carbohydrates have a lesser tendency to store fat.

Habitual Obesity

As I write this and read it to my wife for approval, she reminds me that genetic obesity is often the result of "habitual obesity."

I tell Laura that kids born to obese parents have a 60% chance to grow up obese. She vehemently disagrees." GENETICALLY, they may be burdened, but add to that 60%, the fact that many who are obese overeat, eat the wrong foods, and don't exercise, and you'll quickly realize that a child born to obese parents will have a 90% chance of becoming fat!" So I ask, what is "habitual obesity?"

Says Laura, "It's when your lean grandparents eat all junk food and don't move, and become 20 pounds overweight. Your grandmother gives birth to a son who marries your mom. They mimic the lifestyle of their parents-with inactivity, a high fat and high sugar diet. This causes your parents to become 30 pounds over their ideal weight. When you are born, you follow the dietary habits that are familiar to you and also become fat, probably fatter than your parents who were fatter than their parents."

While we are learning that genetics does play a role in obesity, Laura's point is overeating, making poor choices and inactivity all lead to obesity-even in lean individuals. Some scientists call this "genetics." "I call it bad eating and an environment that supports obesity."

Leptin to the Rescue

There is new evidence that supports the belief that your genetics could be the problem keeping you from achieving your dream body. Researchers of mice have isolated a gene called OB. It is thought that this gene is responsible for weight gain and loss.

When this gene works correctly in laboratory mice, it makes a hormone called leptin. Leptin travels through the blood and signals the brain when the body has stored enough fat. However, if the OB gene is not working properly, rats become lazy. They move around less and gorge themselves with food.

When mice with a genetically skewed OB gene are injected with leptin, they become very active and radically reduce food consumption. Genetically fat rats become trim and even rats that have a normal functioning OB gene lose weight when injected with leptin.

Next, scientists applied the new knowledge to obese humans. Unfortunately, obese humans don't seem to have the defective OB gene, but they do produce leptin. Interestingly, scientists found that obese individuals produce MORE leptin than lean individuals, the opposite of what one would expect. Therefore, scientists are postulating obese humans OVER produce leptin because it may not be binding with its receptor in the brain. The brain may be the next frontier in obesity research.

GLP-1

Another hormone, that may be stimulated by leptin is GLP-1. GLP-1 is also thought to be deficient or defective in obese individuals. GLP-1 works in the brain and in the digestive system. It triggers a person to stop eating by a not fully understood mechanism in the brain. In the digestive tract, it slows down digestion, making you feel "full."

Chapter Fourteen

Supplement and Drink Yourself Thin

Over the years, the market has seen more than its share of pills and drinks that promise fat loss with hardly any effort on your part. Almost every single one of the pills are very overrated and many just don't work at all. However, there are a few nutrients that you can purchase at your local health food store that may be of some help in winning the war on body fat.

Imagine taking a pill that would speed along the fat burning process. Imagine if you could take a nutrient to shed fat faster than with dieting alone. Sound too good to be true?

Let me introduce you to a few nutrients that can be of some help, but understand that taking them alone is probably a waste of time and money. *When combined with a low calorie diet that initiates fat burning*, however, these supplements may enhance fat loss, allowing you to shed more fat than dieting can achieve alone. Moreover, the nutrients that speed fat burning can also help save muscle from being lost.

The theory is simple. Dieting causes the body to shed a combination of fat and some muscle tissue. If fat-burning is enhanced and magnified with the use of a supplement, the body becomes less likely to tap muscle for fuel because it's being adequately fueled by stored body fat.

Let's examine the most popular fat-burning nutrients-what they are, how they work, what they cost, their possible side effects and recommended dosages. I've assigned them an effectiveness rating of 1-5 stars (with five stars meaning the most effective).

Synergisim

You may wish to add one or a combination of these nutrients to a sound exercise program and a calorie controlled diet that's lower in fat and sugar, high in fiber, and makes use of a five meals per day eating plan. Start with one product at a time, allowing at least two weeks to pass before evaluating the results and determining if the product is working. You can then add another nutrient.

Most of these substances seem to complement the effects of one another. For example, many manufacturers make hydroxycitric acid with chromium, as research shows that these two yield much better results together than hydroxycitric acid does alone. A combination of chromium and hydroxycitric acid rates five stars.

Another popular combination is a caffeine-maHuang mixture, since caffeine can prolong the effect of maHuang in the body. (As with many supplements, check with your doctor before trying this combination; some people experience heart palpitations with the maHuang-caffeine mixture.) Fish oils added to chromium will probably have a greater effect than taking chromium or fish oil separately. Taken individually, both will enhance insulin sensitivity; taken together, or adding 25 grams of fiber to the diet, you could expect even better sensitivity. Whatever route you choose, don't subscribe to the mistaken belief that these substances can work magic. Only when combined with sensible eating habits and proper exercise will they expect the desired effect.

The Nutrients

L-Carnitine**

L-Carnitine, a close cousin to amino acids, is found in higher concentrations in organ meats, such as beef liver and beef heart. If organs don't tickle your fancy, try lamb, which is also high in L-Carnitine.

This nutrient was used for 60 years in Europe to treat heart patients with unhealthy amounts of fat in the blood, and was approved in 1986 for use in the United States. Athletes and dieters soon began using it in hopes of aiding fat loss and increased endurance.

Carnitine is a catalyst. When calories are reduced or when a person exercises, fat is tapped as fuel. The body breaks down fat cells to obtain glycerol and fatty acids. Carnitine transports the fatty acids from the blood, across the cell membrane, and into the mitochondrial portion of muscle cells where the fatty acids are burned as fuel. The body can make carnitine from other amino acids and vitamins.

Some research revels that using high amounts of supplemental carnitine can improve aerobic capacity, thereby making exercise easier and promoting additional fat loss by increasing systemic and liver-carnitine stores. In an Italian study published in the <u>European Journal of Applied Physiology</u>, researchers found that cyclists using 2 grams of carnitine significantly increased their maximal oxygen uptake and power output when working at peak intensity. However, other studies conclude carnitine to be helpful only in those who are severely deficient in it.

The theory for dieters is this. If you are freeing up fatty acids with dieting, then your body needs plenty of carnitine to transport fatty acids into muscle cells to be burned as fuel. I feel that Carnitine is helpful, and those who have to follow a low carbohydrate diet will find this nutrient to be especially helpful.

High doses, beyond 3 grams a day, may promote diarrhea in some individuals. Dieters and athletes typically use 1000 mg (one gram) a day before training with weights or before aerobic exercise. These are the peak times when more fat is released from storage to be utilized as fuel.

Recommended Dose: 1000 to 3000 mg a day
Cost: $1 - $3

MaHuang*****

This popular herb (like its principle extract, ephedrine) was originally used to relieve asthma symptoms, achieving its effect by dilating the bronchioles that supply the lungs with oxygen. Another common effect of both maHuang and ephedrine is the stimulation of thermogenesis, a fancy word for heat. Thermogenesis occurs with training, food consumption and the use of certain substances.

Training causes an increase in body temperature, which in turn burns more calories. Each time you eat, your body temperature rises. Some of the calories consumed from a meal are simply dissipated as heat. Protein exerts the strongest thermic effects with carbohydrates second and fat a very distant third.

MaHuang supplements work by releasing the neurotransmitter in the brain called noradrenaline, which exerts a stimulating effect. The body dumps adrenaline from the adrenal glands into the blood and the brain releases noradrenaline; this causes the body temperature to rise and promotes the breakdown of fat cells so that fuel can be obtained to fight, run or perform a large amount of physical work. This is known as the "fight or flight response." Also stimulated by this process is brown fat, which is found surrounding the organs and between the shoulder blades, and is similar to muscle in that it is metabolically active and requires calories. Stimulating brown fat is another way to burn more calories.

In a Danish Study, five women used 25 mg of ephedrine for three months and lost an average of 6 pounds of fat without dieting. Researchers estimated that ephedrine increased the women's daily metabolic rate by 10%. Another study in Obesity Research (1987, vol. 5, pg. 163-168) found that using ephedrine (along with caffeine) allowed obese individuals to lose more fat on average than another group that didn't use ephedrine.

Diabetics and those with thyroid dysfunction, high blood pressure or certain heart problems should not use this product-it can aggravate and intensify pre-existing health conditions. Highly stressed, easily excited and/or chronically nervous individuals should also avoid maHuang. Insomnia, anxiety, or panic attacks may result from doses above the recommended levels.

Recommended Dose: 335 - 670 mg of MaHuang a day (equivalent to 25 - 50 mg of ephedrine). If 670 mg is used, split into two doses of 335 mg each.

Cost: 20 - 40 cents

Fish Oils**

Found in fattier fish like salmon, herring and mackerel, fish oils contain omega-3 fatty acids. Epidemiological studies have conclusively shown that populations that consume copious amounts of fish (such as in the Nordic countries) experience significantly less diabetes than other parts of the world, particularly the United States. The omega-3 fatty aids encourage the receptor sites on muscle to increase insulin sensitivity, allowing the body to release less insulin. In turn, fat storage tends to be limited, and insulin performs its intended job- channeling carbohydrates and amino acids into muscle tissue.

According to Leonard Storlien at the University of Sydney, diets rich in omega-3 fatty acids are effective in overcoming even "very profound whole-body insulin resistance," which is of extreme importance to the overweight.

Recommended Dose: 4000 mg daily, supplying 640 mg of EPA and 480 mg of DHA. This amount can also be found in approximately 4 ounces of salmon.

Cost: 45 cents in supplemental form

Soluble Fiber****

Soluble fiber, common to beans, legumes and oatmeal, can aid fat loss by two distinct mechanisms. First, fiber slows the release of carbohydrates from the stomach into the blood; slowing digestion retards the release of sugar into the blood so that insulin is released at a modified rate. (Lowering insulin levels inhibits fat storage while allowing fat to be used as fuel). Second, fiber works similarly to chromium, vanadyl and fish oils in that it makes muscle tissue receptors more insulin-sensitive; less insulin is thus required to channel carbohydrates into muscle to make muscle glycogen.

An article published in The Lancet (1991, vol. 3, pg. 43 - 45) by Ivellese found that a diet providing 25 to 35 grams a day of a mixture of fibers resulted in lower blood glucose levels in healthy individuals. A review article in Contemporary Nutrition showed that high fiber diets improve glucose sensitivity.

Recommended Dose: 15 - 25 grams daily

Cost: approximately 30 - 60 cents in supplemental form

Caffeine**

Caffeine, a drug found in coffee, tea and chocolate, has long been used as an ergogenic aid by both power and aerobic athletes. Caffeine increases endurance by increasing the breakdown of fat in adipose tissue (body fat). Taken before an aerobic session, it can make the work seem easier, thereby allowing the athlete to train longer and burn more fat and calories. Caffeine also makes the muscle contraction more forceful by promoting greater neurotransmitter release from the nerve at the neuromuscular junction. Adding caffeine to maHuang can significantly enhance and prolong the latter's effect.

Caffeine's ability to increase free fatty acid release from fat cells is hampered when carbohydrates are consumed with coffee, so postpone bagels or muffins if fat loss is your priority. The same precautions that hold for maHuang apply to coffee.

Recommended Dose: 100 - 200 mg before exercise (equal to 2 cups of coffee)

Cost: 10 - 20 cents a cup at home and up to $2 retail

Evening Primrose Oil****

Gamma linolenic acid (GLA), a fatty acid that promotes the formation of hormone like substances call prostaglandins, is found in evening primrose oil. GLA can not be manufactured in the body and is found in very few foods, so it must be supplied either in supplemental form or from the conversion of linoleic acid. The latter process is often compromised by age, alcohol consumption, stress, viral infection or a diet high in saturated fat. Supplemental GLA is therefore the best course.

In lean individuals, GLA can increase the metabolic activity of brown fat. However, obese patients using GLA may see no increase in brown fat activity unless ephedrine or maHuang is added to initiate such activity.

A 1979 study of 38 individuals-all more than 10% above their ideal weights-found that they lost an average of 9 pounds in eight weeks without dieting, by supplementing with 450 mgs of GLA daily. Those with the greatest amount of body fat also lost the most. Furthermore, GLA can release prostaglandins that improve insulin sensitivity, according to an article by Crawford and Haessler published in the JOURNAL OF CLINICAL INVESTIGATION (1993, vol. 4, pg. 111 - 113).

Recommended Dose: 450 mgs of GLA daily, up to 1050 mg daily

Cost: 60 cents - $1.80

Chromium***

Avid readers of health magazines have no doubt noticed advertisements for chromium, a trace mineral often marketed as a fat-burning and muscle building enhancer when used in conjunction with an exercise program.

Chromium seems to be difficult to obtain from the diet, being found in foods that aren't common to the typical American's menu. Brewer's yeast is highest in chromium, with clams, mussels, lobster, mushrooms and oysters being secondary choices. The body tends to excrete chromium during exercise, periods of stress, or when a low-fiber or highly refined diet is consumed.

Using chromium can increase the efficiency of the hormone insulin, which is released after eating carbohydrate-rich foods. Insulin drives sugars derived from these carbohydrates into two places, muscle or fat, both of which have insulin receptors. Chromium makes the receptors on muscle more sensitive, which means that carbohydrates are directed towards muscle rather than fat. When combined with exercise, muscle building is increased and fat storage is (somewhat) inhibited.

Chromium research pioneer Gary Evans, PhD, conducted a six-week double-blind study that showed that weight trainers who supplemented their diet with 200 mcg of chromium daily gained 1 1/2 pounds of muscle. The group that didn't use the supplement gained only 2 ounces of muscle.

In a second study done with football players, Evans' research revealed that those who supplemented with 200 mcg of chromium daily lost 7 1/2 pounds in six weeks, while those who didn't use chromium lost only 2 pounds. These same football players (who consumed an average of 4000 calories daily during training) were all deficient in chromium. Other studies haven't been so positive about the benefits of chromium, although if you are deficient in this nutrient, upping your intake will likely make a significant difference in your training results.

Recommended Dose: 100 -200 mcg daily
COST: 10 - 20 cents

Vanadyl Sulfate**

Vanadyl, another trace mineral with actions similar to chromium, works by MIMICKING the effects of insulin so that muscle uses carbohydrates more easily. As with chromium, a sensitive muscle encourages the body to output less total insulin; when insulin is controlled, the body is more likely to allow fat to be used as fuel. Furthermore, making a muscle more insulin sensitive allows carbohydrates and amino acids to be shunted towards building muscle instead of permitting the carbohydrates to stimulate fat storage.

An increasing amount of research shows that small

quantities of this mineral could be helpful in building muscle and inhibiting fat storage. Anecdotal information has yielded conflicting results. Some claim the mineral improves stamina and enables a person to train with weights with more intensity and effort, therefore burning more calories and adding more lean body mass which increases the metabolism. Others claim the mineral plays severe havoc with blood sugar levels, leading to early fatigue.

Recommended Dose: 5 - 15 mcg a day
Cost: 30 to 90 cents

Hydroxycitric Acid**

Another popular nutrient being used to inhibit fat storage is hydroxycitric acid (HCA). HCA is derived from *Garcinia Cambogia*, which is a fruit native to Africa and Middle Eastern countries. The fruit also goes by the name of tamarind.

HCA can inhibit excess carbohydrates from being stored as body fat. When too many carbohydrates are consumed, or when muscle glycogen stores are full and carbohydrates are eaten, the body releases an enzyme called ATP-citrate lyase, which helps form fat from carbohydrates. HCA can temporarily interfere with this enzyme-making it more difficult to form body fat-and encourages muscle glycogen formation. The latter sends a signal to the brain that diminishes the desire to eat. Effectively forming more liver and muscle glycogen also encourages muscle growth, since glycogen reserves play an integral part in muscle recovery.

Recommended Dose: 750 - 1500 mg per day, split before meals

Cost: approximately 20 - 40 cents

Phenylalanine**

When taken on an empty stomach, this essential amino acid can increase the concentration of the messenger in the brain called noradrenaline. Phenylalanine works as an appetite suppressant in two ways. First, any general stimulation of the brain by noradrenaline will reduce the appetite. Amphetamines, the over-the-counter drug phenylpropanolamine (subtract the "propano" in the middle of the word and you almost get phenylalanine!) and the ultra popular appetite suppressant phentermine all work by similar mechanisms. Of course, the drugs are more powerful than the amino acid. Second, phenylalanine can decrease appetite by releasing more cholecystokinin (CCK) in the brain. CCK is released in small quantities as nutrients pass through, and sends a signal to the brain "indicating" that enough food has been consumed to be satisfied.

Numerous animal studies by Gibbs, Smith and Morley have shown phenylalanine to be a potent appetite suppressant, and a clinical study published in <u>Reviews</u> <u>in</u> <u>Clinical</u> <u>Nutrition</u> (1982, vol. 2, pg. 53 - 59) revealed that *free amino acids* in the gut, especially phenylalanine, can have a profound effect on CCK release in humans.

Any nutrient or drug that can promote the release of adrenaline should be used only under close supervision. The side effects can be similar, though less intense, to those found with maHuang.

Recommended Dose: 100 - 500 mg in the

morning on an empty stomach

Cost: 5 to 20 cents

Water

Water a nutrient? Yes! Many dieters who reduce too fast experience a metabolic downshifting. This occurs because muscle tissue is lost with severe dieting and severe restrictions in energy consumption also trigger fat cells to hoard fat and decrease thermogenesis.

Low calorie diets also decrease the body's output of thyroid hormone which governs the metabolic rate.

Another factor that contributes to the metabolism is water or hydration levels of muscle cells. Water comprises the blood, it is a transporter of nutrients, and it helps to carry waste products from the body. Cutting back on your fluid intake may trigger a slowdown in your metabolism making fat loss harder.

Scientists at the University of Utah administered diuretics to women which caused a loss of water. The weights of the women who used the water excreting pills showed a loss of 2% bodyweight. They also showed a decrease in the resting metabolic rate and a decreased ability to use fat as fuel. Drink up for fat loss!

Chapter Fifteen

Drugs and Weight Loss: 7 With Promise

While diet and exercise are two strong factors that influence obesity, there are several other conditions important in the development of obesity.

Obviously, there are some individuals who respond quickly and successfully to alterations to diet or exercise. What about those who obtain drastically smaller results from diet and exercise? For millions, the answer may be found in drug treatment. The medical profession uses drugs to treat everything from colds, to the flu, to cancer and AIDS, so why not approach obesity as a disease. After all, the obese suffer diabetes, cancer and heart disease at a rate that is significantly higher than the non obese.

Diet and exercise is a proven means to lower body fat levels. The two combined yield better and more permanent results than diet alone or exercise alone. Therefore, a combination of dieting with exercise and pharmaceuticals may be the best way to control obesity. Drug companies sure think so.

Many of the drugs on the market today effect the metabolic system or influence hormones and the nervous system. Manipulating one or all three can effect weight loss or food intake.

The most common and popular drug therapy today includes

A) Drugs that are designed to control how much you eat
B) Drugs that stimulate the brain to make you feel full
C) Drugs that slow food breakdown in the stomach
D) Drugs that interfere with nutrient (carbohydrate and fat) absorption
E) Drugs that increase heat production
F) Drugs that increase lean body mass

Anorectic Drugs

Anorectic drugs work by suppressing the appetite. Obviously, if you eat less food, your weight will decrease. All appetite/anorectic drugs resemble the sympathomimetic amines. Sympathomimetic amines are released in the body as a result of nervous system stimulation. The nervous system has two different parts. They are the parasympathetic and sympathetic systems. At rest, the parasympathetic system tends to dominate and the sympathetic nervous system (SNS) is turned on during exercise and during periods of both physical and mental stress.

The SNS stimulates a cascade of physical reactions that can positively influence metabolism, fat breakdown, and (decreased) food consumption.

Sympathomimetic drugs are relatives to "speed" or amphetamines. Pure amphetamines can promote several effects in humans including a decreased food intake, an increase in mood enhancement, increased SNS stimulation, a change in brain activity and cardiovascular changes. Some effects of amphetamines are beneficial, the decreased food intake and the increased SNS stimulation could lead to calorie expenditure, but the negatives overwhelm the positive benefits. Over stimulation of the brain can lead to dependency and the cardiovascular effects are damaging.

However, there are ways to alter pure amphetamines so the positive effects are retained while the negative effects are either eliminated or more likely, limited.

Phen-Fen

Both phentermine and fenfluramine have been around for years. Both have shown to be moderately successful in decreasing total food consumption. Phentermine works by stimulating the brain which causes a decreased food consumption. While decreasing food consumption will initiate fat loss, phentermine seems to cause more fat loss than can be attributed to a cut in calories alone.

Fenfluramine seem to work by altering the use of the neurotransmitter serotonin. Serotonin is released with a high carbohydrate meal. In lean individuals it seems to stimulate satiety but in the obese, there appears to be some type of defect in serotonin's ability to promote a feeling of being "full." Therefore, a person continues to eat.

Phentermine can increase your energy levels by its stimulating effect on the nervous system, similar to, but much stronger than caffeine from coffee. Being a sympathomimetic, it also releases small amounts of noradrenaline which promotes the "fight or flight" response which, in turn, signals more fat to be broken down to be used as fuel. Due to its stimulating effects, many find it undesirable as there are reports of anxiety, restlessness and insomnia with its use.

Fenfluramine acts as a mild sedative by increasing the release of serotonin. Somehow, increasing or prolonging the effect of this messenger seems to decrease food consumption.

Although these drugs have been on the market for some time, it wasn't until 1992 after a study at the University of Rochester showed a combination of the two appetite suppressing drugs was more effective than the traditional weight loss regimen of low calories and exercise. This study, along with the possibility of unlimited profits from anti-obesity drugs, has caused drug companies to delve further into developing new ways to fight fat.

Redux

Redux, also known as dexfenfluramine, and an offshoot to fenfluramine, is the newest appetite suppressing drug introduced to the marketplace. When it was approved by the FDA, it sent Jenny Craig's stock tumbling down 5 points in one day! Redux is similar to fenfluramine but it is thought it works better, with less side effects, so it can be used for longer periods of time. Some doctors prescribe *Redux* for up to one year while most will try to wean patients off Phen-fen after months.

In a year long study with Redux, 6.4% of subjects using the drug lost 5% or more of their body weight, and more than 20% of the subjects lost at least 15% of their bodyweight. However, a study published in the New England Journal of Medicine (August 29, 1996) reported a rare life-threatening side effect of redux-primary pulmonary hypertension. This condition causes the blood vessels supplying blood to the lungs to become thick and scarred. This can stress the heart forcing it to work harder. Researchers in Europe found those who use redux have a six fold increased chance of experiencing primary pulmonary hypertension and those who use the drug for very long periods of time will be subjecting themselves to a 23 fold increase in risk.

Neither *Redux* or phen-fen are designed for people who have a few pounds to lose or are slightly overweight. First time dieters and those who have less than thirty pounds to lose can radically change body composition and lose fat with the right training and eating program. These pills are not a magic bullet and end all to weight management. The success is due to their ability to decrease the appetite.

Ephedrine

I discussed ephedrine earlier and I feel it is important to further cover this interesting drug as many studies show it to be amazingly successful ingredient to the dieter's arsenal.

Ephedrine is a beta agonist that has been proven to cause an increase in muscle with a loss of fat in animals. Adrenergic receptors that are stimulated by adrenergic agonists (like ephedrine) control the cell's response to stress hormones. Ephedrine stimulates the release of catecholamines in the body. These are stress hormones that act on fat cells by allowing fat to be broken apart to be used as fuel. Ephedrine stimulates the sympathetic nervous system, as does phentermine. The result is a decrease in appetite and an increase in caloric expenditure.

Ephedrine causes calories to be burned in two ways. By stimulating the sympathetic nervous system, it promotes the release of messengers that make a special fat called brown fat more active. Brown fat is located around the organs and between the shoulder blades. It is different from white fat, the fat that is located under the skin and the fat that we all try so hard to lose. Brown fat is similar to muscle tissue in that it is metabolically active. It requires calories. Stimulating it causes more calories to be burned up leading to fat loss. Ironically, lean individuals seem to have brown fat that is more metabolically active than obese individuals. Yet another reason obese stay obese and lean folks stay leaner! The second way ephedrine burns up calories is by increasing dietary induced thermogenesis. Foods cause an increase in heat production which is magnified by ephedrine.

Caffeine prolongs the effect of ephedrine in the body. There are multiple studies that show ephedrine (20 mg a day) combined with caffeine (200 mg) and a reduced calorie diet causes more fat loss than with diet alone. Furthermore, ephedrine and caffeine cause muscle to be spared-so the metabolism stays high. In those who diet alone, some muscle may be lost causing a metabolic slowdown.

Testosterone

Testosterone is the male hormone that dramatically increases upon puberty and declines after the age of 30. It is responsible for secondary sex characteristics of the male-increased facial and body hair and a deepening of the voice.

Testosterone builds muscle. Remember, muscle increases the metabolic rate. While not approved for weight control because it does not work like traditional drugs (decreasing appetite), testosterone could be used to alter the muscle to fat ratio in the body. In a study in The New England Journal of Medicine (July 4, 1996) 40 men were divided into 4 groups. One received 600 milligrams of testosterone a week. The second group received a placebo. The third group received the testosterone plus exercise. The final group received a placebo plus they exercise. The study lasted for ten weeks. Those who took the testosterone experienced a greater increase in muscle than the placebo group. Those who took the testosterone and exercised added the most amount of muscle. Contrary to many reports in the media, none who received the testosterone experienced any hostility or excessive aggression or anger during the ten weeks. Remember, adding just 10 pounds of muscle to a male who has 140 pounds of lean body mass will increase his resting metabolism by

7%.

According to Richard Strauss, M.D. of Ohio State University, severe weight loss programs in male collegiate wrestlers lowers testosterone levels. This serves as a double whammy. I already explained that severe caloric restriction promotes a loss in muscle. Muscle is converted into fuel to make up for a severe caloric loss with very low calorie dieting. Now, we learn testosterone is lowered with very low calorie dieting. This also causes muscle loss further slowing the metabolism.

Growth Hormone

Growth hormone (GH) is released from the pituitary during the first 60 minutes of sleep. It begins to decline after the mid-twenties and is released in smaller and smaller amounts as we age. GH is lipolytic-it burns fat and it promotes an increase muscle weight (lean body mass). Because an increase in fat and a loss of muscle and bone mass is associated with aging, longevity enthusiasts have adopted GH as it's #1 weapon to fight mother nature.

GH can be made in the lab and it is very expensive. Furthermore it requires daily, sometimes twice daily, injections. People use it because they claim to feel better and most like the fat loss/muscle increasing effects. I have read many studies that show an increase in muscle with a decrease in fat with the administration of growth hormone. However, there is an overwhelming amount of evidence that the new muscle is quickly lost and fat regained upon cessation.

L-Dopa

L-Dopa is a prescription amino acid that is used in Parkinson's Disease. It increases the amount of the neurotransmitter in the brain called dopamine, a cousin to the neurotransmitter serotonin (see redux).

Dopamine promotes the release of your own growth hormone from the pituitary. Tests sponsored by the *National Institute on Aging* showed that 500 mgs a day, in pill form, could restore GH levels of men in their sixties to levels that are common to men in their twenties, with no side effects.

Oxandrin

Oxandrin, also known as oxandralone, is made and marketed by a company called Bio-Technology General. Oxandrin is an anabolic hormone, a distant cousin to testosterone. It is similar to testosterone but has been altered to promote an increase in lean body mass without contributing secondary sex alterations that are typical of testosterone. Because the secondary sexual changes in the drug have been altered, this drug may be of use to women.

Right now, this drug is approved to prevent muscle loss in AIDS patients, but I know of one physician in Hollywood who is prescribing it to his clientele for purely cosmetic reasons. The hope is that it will increase muscle and increase fat loss by way of a better metabolism that is associated with more muscle mass.

Appendage 1

Now you have more information and knowledge to continue your quest for a lean body. I am confident that the ideas, theories and tips in this book can help you to radically transform yourself. You have almost everything you need to get going.

The hardest part to losing weight is continuance. For one reason or another, most people are not motivated to stay with a program long enough to see concrete results. My wife thinks she has the answer. It's in her cooking.

She has found that most people can't lose weight because they really hate the taste of low fat and low sugar foods. People miss the junk, the fun stuff, the foods that taste good and make you feel good. Laura always stresses dieting success is correlated to great tasting foods, and since she is the best fat free cook in the world, I thought I would include a few recipes that may help you to stick with your diet.

NO FAT FRENCH FRIES

4 large potatoes (12 ounces)
2 large egg whites beaten
1/4 teaspoon paprika
Non stick cooking spray

1) Cut potatoes 1/2 inch thick in diameter shaped like a fry. 2) Soak in ice cold water for ten minutes. 3) Drain and place on paper towels. 4) Dip potatoes, one at a time, in eggs. 5) Place on top of a thoroughly Pam sprayed non stick cookie sheet. 6) Sprinkle with paprika. Spray potatoes with Pam. 7) Bake at 450° F for 15 minutes, flip and cook another 15 minutes. Serves 4. Calories: 300. Protein: 7. Carbohydrates: 67. Fat: 1.

TUNA BURGERS

1 can white water packed tuna
1 jumbo egg white
1 teaspoon Mrs. Dash
1/2 ounce pancake mix
1 tablespoon chopped onion

1) Drain tuna so little moisture exists. Place in a bowl. 2) Add egg white, pancake mix, spice and onion. Mix together with a fork. 3) Form into 3 inch diameter patties. 4) Grill both sides on a non stick Pam sprayed skillet over a medium heat. Serve on a bun, or alone with no fat french fries. Serves 2. Calories: 120. Protein: 20. Carbohydrates: 12. Fat: 2.

SPICY CHICKEN FINGERS

1 pound chicken breast, cut into small pieces
1 teaspoon cajun spice
1 teaspoon paprika
1/2 cup flour
1 tablespoon Mrs. Dash
2 egg whites

1) Combine spice and flour in a small bowl. 2) Beat egg whites with a fork. 3) Thoroughly spray a non stick pan with Pam. 4) Dip chicken pieces in egg whites then powder in flour mixture. 5) Grill. Serves 4. Calories: 177. Protein: 20. Carbohydrates: 13. Fat: 5.

TURKEY MEATBALLS

1 pound ground turkey breast
2 egg whites
1 small carrot, finely grated
1 stalk green onion, chopped
1 clove garlic
1/2 teaspoon parsley
1/2 teaspoon oregano
2 tablespoons bread crumbs
extra bread crumbs

1) Mix all ingredients. 2) Form into 1 inch diameter balls. Roll into bread crumbs. 3) Pan fry over a low heat in a Pam sprayed non stick skilled. 4) Turn until brown and the center is cooked. Serve with pasta. Serves 8. Calories: 98. Protein: 18. Carbohydrates: 5. Fat: 1.

LAURA'S LO MEIN

4 egg whites
12 ounce box spaghetti
4 tablespoons soy sauce (low sodium)
1/2 cup fat free mayonnaise
1 green onion, chopped

1) Cook spaghetti according to the directions on the box. 2) Store in the refrigerator overnight. 3) Grill onion in a non stick Pam coated skillet. 4) Next, grill the cold spaghetti with the egg whites in the skillet. 5) When the egg turns white, add mayonnaise and soy sauce. 6) Cook another 3 minutes. Serves 5. Calories: 278. Protein: 11. Carbohydrates: 54. Fat: 2.

HONEY MUSTARD CHICKEN

1 pound chicken breast
1/4 cup Worcestershire Sauce
1 tablespoon honey
3 tablespoons mustard
1 tablespoon molasses
1 teaspoon ginger

1) Marinade all ingredients in a bowl overnight. 2) Broil until juicy and tender in an oven broiler set to 450° F. Serves 4. Calories: 140. Protein: 19. Carbohydrates: 7. Fat: 4.

Appendage 2

	Measure	Weight	Calories	Protein	Total Fat	Carbo
BREADS						
Bagels	1	100.0	296	11.0	2.6	56
Brown Bread, with raisins	1/2 slice	45.0	80	2.0	0.0	18
Cinnamon Raisin Bread	1 slice	28.0	80	2.0	1.0	15
Cracked Wheat	1 slice	25.0	66	2.3	0.9	13
English Muffin enriched	1	57.0	130	4.5	1.1	26
Pumpernickel	1 slice	32.0	82	2.9	0.8	15
Roman Meal	1 slice	28.0	70	3.0	1.0	13
Rye	1 slice	25.0	66	2.1	0.9	12
Sourdough	1 slice	28.0	70	3.0	1.0	12
Whole Wheat Bread	1 slice	25.0	61	2.4	1.1	11
CEREALS						
All-Bran	1 oz.	28.0	71	4.0	0.5	21
Alpha Bits	1 C	28.0	110	2.3	0.7	24
Bran, 40%	1 C	47.0	152	5.3	0.8	37
Bran, 100%	1/2 C	28.0	76	3.5	1.4	21
Cheerios	1 1/4 C	28.4	111	4.3	1.5	20
Corn Chex	1 oz. 2	8.0 1	11	2.0	0.1	25
Corn Flakes	1 1/4 C	28.0	110	2.3	0.1	24
Corn Grits, cooked	1C	242.0	146	3.5	0.5	31
Cream of Wheat	1 C	251.0	134	3.8	0.5	28
Grapenuts	1/4 C	28.4	101	3.3	0.1	23
Life	1 oz.	28.0	104	5.2	0.5	20
Malto Meal	1 C	240.0	122	3.5	0.3	26
Nutri-Grain, wheat	3/4 C	8.0	102	2.5	0.3	24
OATMEAL						
Cooked	1 C	234.0	145	6.0	0.4	25
Instant	1 pkg.	177.0	104	4.4	1.7	18
Puffed Rice	1 C	14.0	56	0.9	0.1	13
Puffed Wheat	1 C	14.0	52	2.1	0.2	11
Raisin Bran	1/2 C	28.0	86	2.5	0.5	22
Rolled Oats, dry	1 C	81.0	311	13.0	5.1	54
Roman Meal	3/4 C	181.0	111	4.9	0.7	25
Shredded Wheat	1 lg.	23.6	83	2.6	0.3	19
Toasted Wheat Germ	1/4 C	28.0	108	8.3	3.0	14
Total	1 C	33.0	116	3.3	0.7	26
Wheaties	1 C	28.0	99	2.7	0.5	23
DAIRY						
Blue	1 oz.	28.0	100	6.1	8.2	1
Brie	1 oz.	28.0	95	5.9	7.9	0
Feta	1 oz.	28.0	75	4.0	6.0	1
Parmesan	1 oz.	28.0	111	10.0	7.3	1

	Measure	Weight	Calories	Protein	Total Fat	Carbo
EGGS						
Chicken, Boiled	1	50.0	79	6.1	5.6	1
Chicken, Poached	1	50.0	79	6.0	5.6	1
Chicken, White	1 lge	33.0	16	3.4	0.0	0
Chicken, Whole	1 lge	50.0	79	6.1	5.6	1
EGG SUBSTITUTES						
Country Morning	1/2 C	121.0	173	14.6	12.1	1
Egg Beaters	1/4 C	25	5.0	0.0	1	
FISH						
Bass, baked	4 oz.	113.0	287	23.6	19.4	3
Bluefish, raw	3 oz.	85.0	105	17.0	3.6	0
Carp, cooked	3 oz.	85.0	138	19.4	6.1	0
Clams, steamed	3 oz.	85.0	126	21.7	1.7	4
Cod, baked	3 oz.	85.0	89	19.4	0.7	0
Crab, moist heat	3 oz.	85.0	82	16.5	1.3	0
Flounder, baked	3.5 oz.	100.0	202	30.0	8.2	0
Grouper, broiled	3 oz.	85.0	100	21.1	1.1	0
Haddock, baked	3 oz.	85.0	95	20.6	0.8	0
Halibut, baked	3 oz.	85.0	119	22.7	2.5	0
Kingfish, cooked	3.5 oz.	100.0	255	22.3	13.4	12
Lobster, steamed	3 oz.	85.0	83	17.4	0.5	1
Mackerel, baked	3 oz.	85.0	223	20.3	15.1	0
Mussels, baked	3 oz.	85.0	147	20.2	3.8	6
Ocean Perch, baked	3 oz.	85.0	103	20.3	1.8	0
Orange Roughy, raw	3 oz.	85.0	107	12.5	6.0	0
Oysters, steamed	3 oz.	85.0	117	12.0	4.2	7
Oysters, raw	6 med.	84.0	58	5.9	2.1	3
Pollack, baked	3 oz.	85.0	96	20.0	1.0	0
Salmon, pink, cooked	3 oz.	85.0	118	16.8	5.1	0
Salmon, poached	3 oz.	85.0	157	23.3	6.4	0
Scallops, raw	3 oz.	85.0	75	14.3	0.6	2
Shark, raw	3 oz.	85.0	111	17.8	3.8	0
Shrimp, steamed	3 oz.	85.0	84	17.8	0.9	0
Snapper, baked	3 oz.	85.0	109	22.4	1.5	0
Sole, fillet, frozen	4 oz.	113.0	82	18.0	0.8	1
Squid, Calamari, fried	3 oz.	85.0	149	15.3	6.4	7
Swordfish, baked	3 oz.	85.0	132	21.6	4.4	0
Tuna, water packed	3 oz.	85.0	111	25.1	0.4	0
Tuna, baked	3 oz.	85.0	157	25.4	5.3	0
Whitefish, raw	3 oz.	85.0	114	16.2	5.0	0
FRUIT						
Apple, with skin	1	150.0	81	0.3	0.5	21
Apple, dried	10 rings	64.0	155	0.6	0.2	42
Applesauce, Unsweetened	1 C	244.0	106	0.4	0.1	28
Apricot	3	106.0	51	1.5	0.4	12
Avocado	1	201.0	324	4.0	30.8	15

	Measure	Weight	Calories	Protein	Total Fat	Carbo
Banana	1	114.0	105	1.2	0.6	27
Blueberries	1 C	145.0	82	1.0	0.6	21
Cantaloupe	1 C	160.0	57	1.4	0.4	13
Cherries	1 C	145.0	104	1.7	1.4	24
Dates	10	83.0	228	1.6	0.4	61
Fig	1	65.0	47	0.5	0.2	12
Fruit Cocktail, water packed	1/2 C	122.0	40	0.5	0.1	10
Grapefruit	1/2	120.0	38	0.8	0.1	10
Grapes, Green	1 C	200.0	102	1.0	0.2	27
Honeydew	1/10	129.0	46	0.6	0.1	12
Kiwi	1	76.0	46	0.8	0.3	11
Lemon, raw	1 Med	58.0	17	0.6	0.2	5
Mango	1	207.0	135	1.1	0.6	35
Orange	1	131.0	62	1.2	0.2	15
Papaya	1	304.0	117	1.9	0.4	30
Peach	1	87.0	37	0.6	0.1	10
Pear	1	166.0	98	0.7	0.7	25
Pineapple	1 C	155.0	77	0.6	0.7	19
Plum	1	66.0	36	0.5	0.4	9
Prune	10	84.0	201	2.2	0.4	53
Raisins, packed	1 C	165.0	488	5.3	0.8	0
Strawberries, fresh	1 C	149.0	45	0.9	0.6	10
Tangerine	1	84.0	37	0.5	0.2	9

MEATS

BEEF

	Measure	Weight	Calories	Protein	Total Fat	Carbo
Flank Steak	4 oz.	114.0	222	21.9	14.3	0
Ground Beef, Lean	4 oz.	113.0	298	28.0	20.9	0
Heart	3 oz.	85.0	148	24.5	4.8	0
Liver	4 oz.	113.0	183	27.6	5.5	4
Porterhouse Steak	4 oz.	114.0	322	20.0	26.4	0
Round Steak	4 oz.	114.0	273	22.0	19.9	0
Sirloin Steak	4 oz.	114.0	295	20.7	22.9	0
T-Bone Steak	4 oz.	114.0	337	29.0	24.0	0
Tenderloin	4 oz.	114.0	308	29.0	20.4	0

LAMB

	Measure	Weight	Calories	Protein	Total Fat	Carbo
Leg of lamb	4 oz.	114.0	211	32.0	7.6	0
Chops	4 oz.	114.0	350	25.5	26.7	0
Shoulder	4 oz.	114.0	315	27.7	22.0	0

VEAL

	Measure	Weight	Calories	Protein	Total Fat	Carbo
Cutlet	4 oz.	114.0	170	18.1	10.3	0
Rump Roast	4 oz.	114.0	143	17.0	7.8	0

LUNCHEON MEAT/SAUSAGE

	Measure	Weight	Calories	Protein	Total Fat	Carbo
Turkey, breast meat	1 slice	21.0	23	4.7	0.3	0

	Measure	Weight	Calories	Protein	Total Fat	Carbo

POULTRY
CHICKEN

	Measure	Weight	Calories	Protein	Total Fat	Carbo
Capon, skin, roasted	3.5 oz.	100.0	229	29.0	11.7	0
Dark w/ skin, roasted	3.5 oz.	100.0	253	26.0	15.8	0
Dark w/o skin, roasted	3.5 oz.	100.0	205	27.4	9.7	0
Light w/ skin, roasted	3.5 oz.	100.0	222	29.0	10.9	0
Light w/o skin, roasted	3.5 oz.	100.0	173	30.9	4.5	0
Whole w/o skin, stewed	3.5 oz.	100.0	177	27.3	6.7	0

TURKEY

	Measure	Weight	Calories	Protein	Total Fat	Carbo
Dark w/o skin, roasted	3.5 oz.	100.0	187	28.6	7.2	0
Light w/o skin, roasted	3.5 oz.	100.0	157	29.9	3.2	0

SAUCES

	Measure	Weight	Calories	Protein	Total Fat	Carbo
Barbeque	1 T	16.0	12	0.3	0.3	2
Catsup	1 T	15.0	16	0.3	0.1	4
Heinz Catsup	1 T		18	0.2	0.0	4
Heinz Chili Sauce	1 T		17	0.2	0.0	4
Heinz 57 Sauce	1 T		15	0.4	0.2	3
Horseradish	1 T	15.0	6	0.2	0.0	1
Mustard, Yellow	1 T	5.0	4	0.2	0.2	0
Mustard, Brown	1 t	5.0	5	0.3	0.3	0
Open Pit, Hickory	1 T	18.0	22	0.1	0.2	5
Pizza Sauce	1/4 C	60.0	40	0.0	2.0	5
Prego	1/4 C	113.0	136	1.9	5.6	20
Spaghetti Sauce, canned	1 C	249.0	272	4.5	11.9	40
Tamari, Soy Sauce					0.1	3
Worcestershire	1 T	11				

VEGETABLES

	Measure	Weight	Calories	Protein	Total Fat	Carbo
Beets, cooked	1/2 C	85.0	26	0.9	0.0	6
Broccoli, raw	1 C	88.0	24	2.6	0.3	5
Carrot, raw	1 med.	72.0	31	0.7	0.1	7
Cauliflower, raw	1 C	100.0	24	2.0	0.2	5
Celery, raw	1 stalk	40.0	6	0.3	0.1	2
Corn, yellow, cooked	1/2 C	82.0	89	2.7	1.1	21
Cucumber, raw	1 C	104.0	14	0.6	0.1	3
Eggplant, raw	1 C	82.0	22	0.9	0.1	5
Green Beans, cooked	1/2 C	62.0	22	1.2	0.2	5
Lettuce, Iceberg	1 C	75.0	10	0.7	0.1	2
Lettuce, Romaine	1 C	56.0	8	0.9	0.1	1
Mixed Vegetables, frozen	1/2 C	91.0	54	2.6	0.1	12
Mushrooms, raw	1 C	70.0	18	1.5	0.3	3
Okra, cooked	1/2 C	80.0	25	1.5	0.1	6
Onions, Mature, raw	1 C	160.0	54	1.9	0.4	12
Peas, frozen	1/2 C	80.0	63	4.1	0.2	11
Pepper, Green, raw	1/2 C	50.0	12	0.4	0.2	3

	Measure	Weight	Calories	Protein	Total Fat	Carbo
POTATOES						
Raw w/o skin	1	112.0	88	2.3	0.1	20
Baked w/ skin	1 lg.	202.0	220	4.7	0.2	51
SQUASH						
Acorn, cooked, mashed	1/2 C	122.0	41	0.8	0.1	11
Spaghetti, cooked	1/2 C	78.0	23	0.5	0.2	5
Sweet Potato, baked	1	114.0	118	2.0	0.1	28
Water Chestnuts, canned	1/2 C	70.0	35	0.6	0.0	9

SOURCES

Aceto, Chris (1996) Championship Bodybuilding. Adamsville, TN: Fundco Printers.

Aceto, Chris (1993) The Health Handbook. Adamsville, TN: Fundco Printers.

Bursztein, Elwyn, Alkanazi and Kinney (1989) Energy, Metabolism, Indirect Calorimetry and Nutrition. Baltimore, MD: Williams and Wilkins.

Kapit, Macey and Meisami (1987) The Physiology Coloring Book. NY, NY: Harper Collins Publishers, Inc.

Page, Hardin and Melnik (1989) Nutritional Assessment and Support. Baltimore, MD: Williams and Wilkins.

Pearson and Shaw (1986) The Life Extension Weight Loss Program. Garden City, NY: Doubleday and Company, Inc.

Rhoades and Pflanzer (1992) Human Physiology. Orlando, FL: Saunders College Publishing.

Stunkard, Albert (1980) Obesity. Philadelphia, PA: WB Saunders Company.

ORDER FORM

A   CHAMPIONSHIP BODYBUILDING:
The know-how and strategies to build muscle
without adding bodyfat $24.95

B   THE HEALTH HANDBOOK:
An easy-to-read guide to total health $19.95

C   A TASTE OF CLUB CREAVALLE:
335 low-fat recipes. Rated 4 stars by several cooking magazines.........$24.95

D   THE LITE LIFESTYLE:
150 Fat-Free Sugar-Free recipes.
A favorite for athletes and diabetics $19.95

E   EVERYTHING YOU NEED TO KNOW ABOUT FAT LOSS:
Great companion to Championship Bodybuilding............................$19.95

F   UNDERSTANDING BODYBUILDING NUTRITION & TRAINING:
Q & A - Addressing hundreds of the most asked questions $19.95

SEND ORDER TO:
**Club Creavalle, P.O. Box 557, Old Orchard Beach, ME 04064
OR Call Now 1-207-934-7812
Visit our Website at www.clubcreavalle.com**

ITEM	QTY.	PRICE	TOTAL
		SUB TOTAL	
ADD $2 PER ITEM FOR S&H			
		TOTAL	

Name _____

Address_____

City, State, Zip: _____

Card No.: _____Expiry Date: _____

Signature: _____Phone:_____

❑ Check   ❑ Money Order   ❑ VISA   ❑ MasterCard